Advance praise for

The Ins and Outs of POOP

A Guide to Treating Childhood Constipation

This is a marvelous book that desperately needed to be written. It is written in simple straightforward language, but all the information is there. Functional constipation is a condition where knowledge really is power. I can't tell you how often, in working with parents, I've heard "He can't be constipated. He goes every day." There is so much misunderstanding around this condition. Dr. DuHamel does everyone a great service in demystifying the whole process of functional constipation and then breaking down the solution into simple steps that lead to recovery. This book should be of great help to parents, children and those that serve them.

• ***Robert Telzrow, MD, Pediatrician***

Chronic constipation and toilet resistance in children is a major source of concern and frustration to parents. To the pediatrician and family physician, the care of this condition demands extensive time in the office and on the phone. Dr. DuHamel has created a clear, logical and effective guide to help both the parent and practitioner treat and correct this challenging problem. *The Ins and Outs of Poop* is not just another toilet training book. It is a unique and positive manual for dealing with one of pediatrics most common and least discussed problems.

• ***Gary B. Spector, MD, Pediatrician***

After dealing with GI issues for six long years, we were shocked to see such a quick turnaround. In just a small period of time on this program, our son started pooping regularly once a day. He has been happier and more confident, which makes our lives much less stressful. It has been a miracle! • ***Stiroh Lang, Parent***

The Ins and Outs of Poop provides clinicians with a manual for how to deal with the unfamiliar world of childhood functional constipation. As Dr. DuHamel explains, issues related to withholding or stool incontinence can be misinterpreted as being related to an emotional disturbance. Clinicians and parents will learn that withholding and stool incontinence are not willful behaviors and, in most cases, the child is not intending to be defiant. This book sheds light on the etiology of functional constipation as well as effective treatment strategies. Parents no longer need to feel hopeless about their child's toileting issues. I have used the six-step program with many of my patients who have sought treatment for functional constipation. I can attest to its efficacy and the relief parents and children feel when this problem no longer dominates their lives.

• ***Lauren Silvers, PhD, Clinical Psychologist***

Constipation is a problem that presents often in my clinical pediatric practice. It is extremely frustrating for parents, children and, at times, providers. Dr. DuHamel's book is an excellent resource that covers all aspects of this issue. It is concise and well organized.
In my 30 years of practice, I have rarely come across a book that is so thorough and user friendly. I envision using this book frequently when working with these families. I would strongly recommend *The Ins and Outs of Poop* as an invaluable addition to nurse practitioners' and physicians' personal libraries.

• ***Nancy Lockett, ARNP, MS, Maternal Child Health***

The Ins and Outs of Poop is a one stop resource for pediatricians, clinicians, and parents dealing with children suffering from constipation. Dr. DuHamel provides a proven treatment blue print. He details the underpinnings of constipation, anticipates potential roadblocks that can occur in treatment, and offers strategies as to how to successfully navigate them. I have incorporated the six-step approach into my practice and find it to be an essential tool for educating parents, successfully treating the child's constipation, and reducing family stress. *The Ins and Outs of Poop* is the definitive guide for addressing childhood constipation.

• ***Paul S. Lapuc, PhD, Clinical Psychologist***

Before we met Dr. Tom, accidents, hidden underwear, discussions about whether or not he had really gone to the bathroom and bed-wetting were all part of daily life for our almost nine year old son. He was initially unenthusiastic about talking to yet another doctor but being an active participant in deciding how much medicine he needed and what he could do to control his bedwetting really helped him feel more in control. Now, just seven months later, my son no longer soils his underwear or wets the bed and he can do sleep-overs without fear of accidents. We have also seen a huge boost in his self esteem. His success on Dr. Tom's program has been truly amazing.

• ***John Brooks, Parent***

A significant number (approximately one third to one half) of adults with functional gastrointestinal disorders report having abdominal pain and bowel problems as children. This book will be very useful to parents and children in learning strategies early in life that may reduce or prevent the long term impact of functional constipation in their adult years.

• ***Margaret Heitkemper, PhD, RN, FAAN***
Professor and Chair, Biobehavioral Nursing and Health Systems
University of Washington School of Nursing

This excellent little book is packed with useful information, logically presented, and accompanied by many helpful tables and illustrations. Even though, as a general internist, my practice did not include children with chronic constipation, I certainly found much in the book's presentation of diagnostic and therapeutic principles that would be applicable to the treatment of adults with chronic constipation. Many readers, including health care providers and parents of children with chronic constipation, will find *The Ins and Outs of Poop* to be a valuable resource.

• ***James Findlay Wallace, MD , MACP, General Internist***
Former Director, Medicine Residency Program
University of Washington School of Medicine

The Ins and Outs of POOP

A Guide to Treating Childhood Constipation

Includes a Six-Step Program for Kids Who Withhold or Soil

THOMAS R. DUHAMEL, PHD

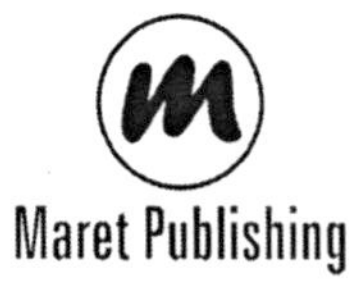

Maret Publishing
Seattle, Washington

Maret Publishing
P.O. Box 25606
Seattle, Washington 98165

Illustrations and Cover Design: Kev Brockschmidt

ISBN: 978-0-9854969-1-3
Library of Congress Control Number: 2012906800

Printed in the United States of America
First Edition
First Printing

Where there is understanding
there is no blame.

• *David Gurteen*

Dedicated to families struggling with childhood constipation

Table of Contents

PART 2 - TREATING CONSTIPATION

PART 3 - GUIDE FOR PROVIDERS

Acknowledgments

This book would not have been written without the encouragement of my family, friends, and colleagues and the many parents and children who have taught me about the heartaches and frustration of living with childhood constipation. I am especially indebted to those parents who graciously took the time to write their stories for inclusion in this book.

I particularly want to thank Kev Brockschmidt for his creative illustrations and layout and Melanie Austin for her expert editing. Most of all, I want to give special thanks to my editor-in-chief and ever-patient wife, Martha, to my children, Jennifer and Tom, and to my granddaughter, Maret, who provided all the inspiration I needed to make it through the ins and outs of writing this book.

Foreword

Effective treatment for functional constipation has been a problem because clinicians and parents feel awkward and embarrassed about *poo* and pooping in our culture. Of course, children learn those attitudes from their parents. It is possible to avoid months or years of worry and discomfort by attending to painful or scary aspects of pooping immediately. The longer a child suffers with functional constipation, the longer it takes to treat. The shorter the time to treatment, the quicker functional constipation resolves.

Functional constipation is a common problem. No testing is necessary or desirable. It is the most common problem to be evaluated and treated by pediatric gastroenterologists. If your constipated child is in a classroom with 29 other first graders, chances are good that there is another student in class with the same problem. It is also probable that because of their shame, they share this information with no one. Each child believes that this problem is their's alone.

When I walk into the room to evaluate a new patient with functional constipation, the toddler is hiding behind the parent, tightly clinging to an arm or leg; the seven-year-old has his head down and states that he does not know why he is seeing a clinician. The toddler is afraid; the school-aged child has a feigned nonchalance. The first thing I say to the child and parent is that I will not do anything that hurts during the visit. Sometimes that allows the child to relax and pay attention to words that can change their lives. I know what is wrong: it's called functional constipation. It is not dangerous. It always goes away when the child decides to allow the poo to come out. The impaction is not the bowel obstruction. The bowel obstruction is in the mind that controls the pelvic floor muscles. There is a lot we can do to help the child choose to let the poo come out. We can always assure painless pooping.

This book contains all the "secrets" a clinician or parent needs to know about functional constipation in childhood. Readers will be empowered to assist their children in ridding them of a sticky problem. I hope that this book finds its way into every primary care clinician's office, and to parents who do not have a clinician who is comfortable with poo.

Paul E. Hyman, MD
Professor of Pediatrics, Louisiana State University
Chief, Pediatric Gastroenterology, Children's Hospital of New Orleans

Dr. Hyman chaired the Pediatric ROME II Working Team and co-chaired the Infants/Toddlers ROME III Working Team, committees charged by the Rome Foundation with developing symptom-based criteria for the diagnosis and treatment of childhood functional bowel disorders.

Preface

My interest in childhood constipation began when I was on the staff of a large pediatric hospital in Seattle and assigned to an outpatient clinic for children with functional constipation, or *encopresis.*

Working with pediatricians, gastrointestinal (GI) specialists, nurses and nurse practitioners, I learned that the successful treatment of functional constipation requires a combination of medical and behavioral interventions. I also learned that I enjoyed working with families who came to the clinic looking for answers. The parents were highly motivated to resolve their child's problem, but success was seldom easy and never instantaneous. These families challenged all of my professional skills and their successes gave me much personal and professional satisfaction.

For the past 30 years I have continued to work with encopretic children in my private practice. Through further study and clinical experience, I know more now about functional constipation than I ever could have imagined. What has not changed is my desire to lessen the misery of families struggling with this condition.

This book is intended as both a resource and a guide for parents and health care providers including pediatricians, GI specialists, family practice physicians, nurse practitioners, nurses, and clinical psychologists. Whether you are a parent or a healthcare professional, this book contains all the information you need to diagnose, treat, and prevent functional constipation.

Introduction

ABOUT THIS BOOK

This book is for children like April. April is an almost 5-year-old girl who was referred by her pediatrician because of severe constipation. From the moment she first walked into my office, it was clear that April was struggling to hold back her stool. Every few minutes, she would get a strained look on her face, stand up straight, bend her upper body slightly forward and squeeze her knees together. When her mother pleadingly suggested that she go to the bathroom, April grimaced and stated emphatically, "I feel fine. I do not have to poop!"

April has a little known but increasingly common problem for children called *functional constipation.* In more severe cases, functional constipation causes children to become *stool incontinent* or to "soil" or defecate in their clothing. A medical term for stool incontinence is encopresis. However, even though encopresis is just one symptom of functional constipation, many pediatric healthcare providers and parents have come to use the term in place of functional constipation. For simplicity, functional constipation is used in this book to encompass issues pertaining to children who are stool incontinent and those who are not.

Functional constipation

Functional constipation follows a fairly predictable course. It usually begins with an uncomfortable or painful bowel movement which can occur as early as the first few months of life. Following one or more painful bowel movements, a child begins to withhold stool to avoid pain whenever he or she feels the need to "poop." This is exactly what April was doing in my office. Initially, April's decision to withhold stool was voluntary, but as her uncomfortable bowel movements continued, her withholding became what psychologists call a *conditioned avoidance response*. It was no longer intentional because it happened automatically. In other words, the act of withholding developed into a habit which continues even when April's bowel movements no longer hurt.

Withholding causes stool to be retained in the rectum. Think of the rectum as a round muscle with an empty space in the center, like a small balloon. As the rectum stretches to accommodate increasing amounts of stool, it periodically contracts in an effort to expel the excess stool. These repeated contractions cause the walls of the rectum to get thicker and stronger. As the rectum gets stronger, however, it also becomes less sensitive and less adept at signaling the need to poop. This often leads to stool incontinence. Moreover, once the rectum is stretched, it remains stretched for a long time even after the excess stool has been removed. While the onset of functional constipation can occur quickly, breaking the habit of withholding and giving the rectum sufficient time to shrink back to its normal size can take many months or years.

Collaboration

In order to treat functional constipation effectively, parents and pediatric healthcare providers must collaborate. The degree of collaboration required distinguishes this particular relationship from the more typical patient-provider relationship. Parents and providers work diligently as a treatment team over an extended period of time to manage and resolve the problem. This book, written for both parents and providers, is meant to encourage frequent communication and sharing of important information throughout the course of a child's treatment. Such communication will increase the likelihood of success, decrease the length of treatment, and enhance parent-child and patient-provider relationships during the treatment process.

Six-Step Program

There are six steps that must be followed to effectively manage functional constipation. Your pediatric healthcare provider will get you started, but you will be the one who provides the bulk of your child's care. The six steps are:

1. Educate the family
2. Empty the rectum
3. End withholding
4. Shrink the rectum
5. Withdraw laxatives
6. Remain vigilant

Each step will be explained in more detail in chapter 8.

From beginning to end, the course of treatment for functional constipation is stressful for everyone including healthcare providers. In my sessions with parents, I tell them that I am their coach and cheerleader. My job is to help them perform to the best of their ability, but they are the ones who have to carry out the game plan. Success requires that parents and providers know not only what to do but also how to do it. As difficult as it may be, parents and providers need to maintain a positive attitude. A negative or punitive attitude will only make the problem worse.

To stay positive, you need to:

1. Be patient!
2. Try not to be judgmental.
3. Remember that withholding and stool incontinence are not intentional.

How to use this book

If your child is not mildly or severely constipated, you may want to find out how to prevent occasional constipation from becoming functional constipation in the future. I suggest that you read chapter 2 first and then chapter 5. Chapter 2 is the story of one mother's struggle with encopresis. Chapter 5 explains how functional constipation can be prevented by quickly and correctly treating occasional constipation.

If your child is severely constipated, you may be eager to go directly to chapter 8 which includes the Six-Step Program for treating functional constipation. However, if you do so, you will quickly see that you cannot effectively implement the Six-Step Program without the information contained in chapters 3–7 and 9–16. Functional constipation is a complex problem. The more you and your child know about the problem the better the outcome will be.

My Child Is Not Constipated

1

Why should I read this book?

Occasional or mild constipation, the kind that comes and goes in a week or two, is very common in children. However, more than 20% of children who have occasional constipation go on to develop a more severe type of constipation known as functional constipation.[1] Functional constipation occurs when children do not sense the need to defecate. Some of these children accidentally soil in their underwear, which causes them and their family shame and embarrassment. Functional constipation is not a disease but it does cause serious physical and emotional problems which can be prevented by knowing what to do when your child develops mild or occasional constipation.

Children at risk for constipation

Most children develop occasional constipation for reasons that are right in front of their parents' eyes. Children in the United States are increasingly sedentary and overweight. Fast food has become the food of choice. Like most adults, children rarely consume enough fiber. As a result of all these factors, children are more likely to become constipated.

For many children, computers, televisions, and hand-held video games have taken the place of active and imaginary play.

Increasingly, children choose to stay inside rather than go outside to play. Physical exercise (walking and running) contributes to stool motility and the frequency of bowel movements. If your child does not get enough physical exercise, he or she is more likely to become constipated.

Some children get so engrossed or hyper-focused while playing "screen" games that they ignore the need to go to the bathroom. The more they do this, the more their stool dries and hardens, making it more difficult for them to have a bowel movement whenever they do decide to go to the bathroom. If your child spends a lot of time absorbed in screen play, he or she is much more likely to become constipated.

One key factor in promoting regularity in adults and children alike is a diet high in fiber. Unfortunately, children often reject whole grain cereals and bread, leafy greens, vegetables, and fruit in favor of sugary, refined cereals, snack foods, and greasy fast food. Instead of snacking on fruit or veggies, they are more likely to be eating packaged chips or cookies, which tend to be low in fiber, but high in fat.

Signs of occasional and functional constipation

You can find out if your child has occasional or functional constipation by reviewing Table 1.1 and by completing the Childhood Constipation Questionnaire in the Appendix.

Table 1.1 Signs of Occasional and Functional Constipation

SIGNS OF OCCASIONAL AND FUNCTIONAL CONSTIPATION			
BOWEL HABITS	NORMAL	OCCASIONAL CONSTIPATION	FUNCTIONAL CONSTIPATION
Frequency	4-10 bowel movements per week	4-5 bowel movements per week	3 or fewer bowel movements per week
Shape and surface of stool	"Banana" or "log" with smooth surface	"Sausage" with cracks	Sausage/ball/pellet-shaped stools with cracked, lumpy surfaces
Color of stool	"Golden Brown" to medium brown	Dark to very dark brown	Dark to almost black color
Hard to "push"	Never or rarely	Occasionally	Frequently
Uncomfortable or painful to pass stool	Never or rarely	Occasionally	Frequently
Habitual stool withholding	Never	Never	Always
Soils underwear	Never	Never	Often

Chapter Notes

1. Loening-Baucke, V. (2007). Prevalence rates for constipation and faecal and urinary incontinence. *Archives of Disease in Childhood*, 92, 486–489.

One Mother's Story

2

Unless your child, or another child you know, has struggled with functional constipation (encopresis), you may find this problem difficult to understand. Encopresis is a confusing and frustrating problem. Put yourself in this mother's shoes and try to imagine how you would react in her situation.

A Tale of Dead Ends

The IKEA playroom attendant put a bracelet on Sarina and handed me the pager that would buzz when our time was up. I took her shoes off, showed her where the potty was, gave her a kiss and watched her bound into the playroom. She headed straight for the giant ball pit and leapt in.

It was too perfect. I felt a little giddy. Sarina was safe and happy, and I had a full hour to myself. I couldn't wait to start strolling through the store tossing tea lights, picture frames and pretty baskets into my bag.

After about 30 minutes the pager went off. Something was wrong. I hurried to the playroom. Sarina was standing by the desk with a worried look. There was no mistaking the foul smell "Your daughter didn't make it to the bathroom," whispered the IKEA attendant. "We have to close the ball room for the day."

I quietly led Sarina away, cleaned her up and headed home. Though she had been out of diapers for well over a year, she almost never pooped in the potty. I had no reason to think she would stay clean at IKEA. I wanted to believe that this would magically be the day she'd get it right.

Sarina would soon be four years old. I watched friends with children the same age as they slowly reclaimed the freedoms of their pre-child lives—going out with friends, getting back to the gym, taking classes. While their worlds were getting bigger, mine was getting smaller. Three-year-olds who aren't potty trained can't be dropped off for play dates, parties, camps or classes. I was with Sarina all day, every day. I desperately needed a break.

Sarina's toileting troubles were taking over our lives. She had no problem urinating in the potty but went days without moving her bowels. When she did have a bowel movement, it was rarely in the bathroom. Sometimes the bowel movements were shockingly large. Cleaning her up was often a horrible, disgusting mess. It felt surreal to be wringing out underpants over the toilet for a child who clearly knew how to take herself to the bathroom.

For more than two years I thought I was locked in a power struggle over potty training. I tried everything I could think of and regularly consulted our family doctor for help. Sticker charts, prizes, potty-sits after meals. Nothing worked. Friends and family members were supportive, but it was always stressful being around other people who, like me, suspected I must have done something horribly wrong to have a child who was regularly soiling herself.

The situation became worse as kindergarten closed in. We started noticing that Sarina not only refused to take herself to the bathroom to poop but also tried her best not to poop at all. It was painful to watch as she clamped her knees together and bent over, working as hard as she could to keep her poop from coming out. When a little would escape, as often happened, it was dark and foul smelling. Even then Sarina would never admit she needed to be cleaned up and never asked to be cleaned. One afternoon after she had dirtied her underpants, I decided to wait and see how long it would take her to come to me for help. Hours passed and the stench was awful. I was in despair.

Ironically, we became aware of some neighbors with an 8-year-old girl who was coming home from school with dirty underpants. Her mother had started putting panty-liners in them. Her parents were miffed because their daughter didn't seem to care that her underpants were dirty or notice the smell. Her mom told me about a special nurse they were seeing who advised them to give their daughter a laxative and chart a schedule of potty-sits.

"I can't sign her up for Girl Scout camp this summer or let her go to sleepovers," said her mom. "It's awful, and I don't know what to do," she confided. I listened and offered words of encouragement. Looking back, I can't believe I never made a connection between the behaviors of the two girls. Their daughter's troubles seemed nothing like my daughter's refusal to potty train.

I continued to try to "potty train" Sarina. I tried getting angry about her poopy messes. I tried ignoring the problem. I tried being encouraging and positive. I tried making her feel guilty. It was exhausting. Finally, with kindergarten just a few days away, I recalled our neighbor's mention of the special nurse they had seen and called. The nurse on the other end of the line curtly asked me a few questions. I heard myself saying yes, there's dark, chalky, super stinky skid marks in her underpants. Yes, she tries to hold in her poop as hard as she can. Yes, she sometimes makes giant BMs.

"Your daughter has encopresis," the nurse said. "She needs to be treated. Our wait list is three months long, and we don't take

your insurance. Call us in November." She hung up.

Finally there was a name for Sarina's problem—encopresis. I had no idea what encopresis was all about, but I did know I couldn't wait three months to get help. We were in crisis. Finding treatment became a full-time job. I went online and learned that Sarina's repeated "withholding" had caused her stool to dry out and harden and her colon to enlarge. Her bowel was blocked. Soft, unformed stool was leaking out into her underpants. It was black and fetid. As was the case with Sarina, children with encopresis lose sensation in their rectum and can't feel the stool seeping out. They may also be in total denial of their condition. Getting Sarina "cleaned out" was my first priority.

I rushed Sarina to our family doctor. "We don't do enemas," the nurse explained. "I don't treat encopresis," stated the doctor. "She needs a psych evaluation and something like Prozac. Good luck." That was dead end number one. More research led us to a children's hospital's GI unit. An x-ray revealed what we expected. "She's full of poop," the nurse said. She gave Sarina an enema. "But what's going to prevent us from ending up right back here in a few weeks?" I questioned. "None of our psychologists are taking new patients, sorry," was the reply. Sure enough, we were back in a few weeks.

I scrolled through the insurance company's long list of family therapists and child psychologists. Only a few were taking new patients. I called them and in one case went for a short interview. None had any experience with encopresis.

Eventually Sarina started seeing a therapist specializing in play-therapy who claimed to have had some success helping children with her problem. After just a few visits, however, it was obvious that she couldn't help us. In the meantime, Sarina was backed up all over again and soiling at school. Her teacher would smell something bad, Sarina would be sent to the office, and I would be called in to clean her up. These were sad times. I would find Sarina alone in the nurses office, sobbing. After cleaning her up and wiping her tears, I would send her back to class.

Sarina clearly understood that if she held in her poop, some would leak out at school and she'd suffer terrible embarrassment when someone noticed the smell. Yet day after day she continued to withhold. It was baffling. I felt totally helpless and couldn't believe how seemingly impossible it was to find effective treatment. The hospitals would treat the physical symptoms, but clearly there was a huge emotional/mental component that mystified everyone.

It had been months since we had spoken to our neighbors, but my husband, Jim, called them to ask if they had found anyone to help their daughter with her condition, which we now knew was encopresis. They gave us the name of a child psychologist who specialized in treating this very condition and told us how well their daughter was doing. I called, certain I'd be told that Dr. DuHamel wasn't taking new patients. After a brief conversation with him, we had an appointment. Finally, after years of dead ends, we had help.

Though it has been years since her recovery, when Sarina runs into the bathroom shouting, "I have to poop," I still feel an enormous sense of relief. The overwhelming frustration of not knowing how to make Sarina better was devastating. Being out from under the pain and being able to truly delight in every cartwheel, costume and misspelled poem is a blessing.

• ***Sharon J.***

This is just one example of the lengthy search that parents often undertake in order to find help for their children. If your child is severely constipated, this book will provide you with most of the answers you have been looking for. You may not like the answers, but at least you will know what your child's problem is and how to manage it.

How Food Becomes Poop

3

The gastrointestinal (GI) tract

The process of creating stool begins with digestion. Think of your body's digestive system as a food processor that works day and night to transform the food you eat into the basic elements you need to live. Digestion takes place in the *upper* gastrointestinal tract, often referred to as the upper GI which includes your stomach and your small intestine. Your *lower* GI, your large intestine, manages the waste left over from digestion and is responsible for converting the waste into stool and removing it from your body.[1]

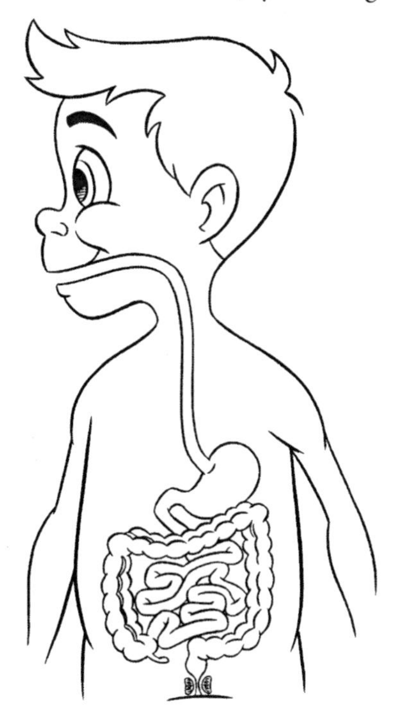

Figure 3.1 GI Tract

Tubes and waves

The GI tract consists of a series of hollow organs joined in long twisting tubes that begin at the mouth and end at the anus. The entire tract is approximately 30 feet long and contains an inner layer of smooth muscle that works within and between organs to move digesting food and waste. The smooth muscle contracts to create a narrowing and then propels the narrow portion forward. This muscle action, which is called *peristalsis*, looks like an ocean wave traveling slowly through the muscle (Figure 3.2). After you swallow, peristalsis is involuntary: you have no control over your food until it reaches your anus as stool, at which time you can voluntarily decide to let it out or not.[2]

Figure 3.2. Peristalsis

The tsunami reflex

The gastrocolic reflex refers to vigorous peristaltic activity, or *mass movements*, primarily in the transverse and descending sections of the colon in response to stretching in the walls of the stomach. The mass movements are like a tsunami reflex (Figure 3.3) that "kicks in" within as little as 15 minutes following a meal or a snack. It is as if the body warns the rectum that more waste is heading its way from above and, therefore, should empty itself to prevent a backup. Mass movements appear to follow a circadian rhythm; they are significantly greater between 6 a.m. and 2 p.m. than between 4 p.m. and 4 a.m. The gastrocolic reflex plays a major role in the management of functional constipation.

Figure 3.3 Tsunami Reflex

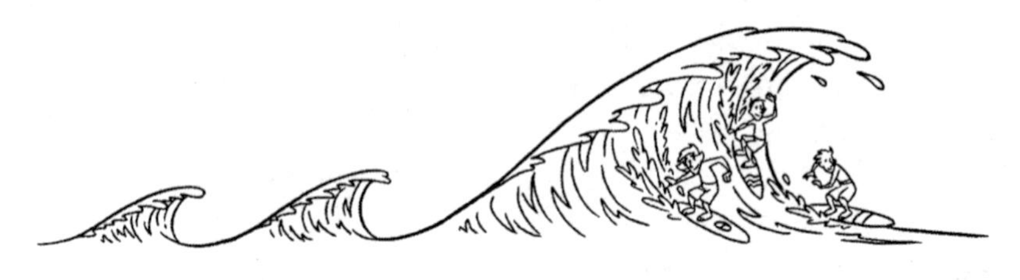

Fiber beats meat

Many children and even some adults believe that the last food they eat is the first stool that comes out. In fact, it can take more than 72 hours before the food you eat passes through your anus. The time it takes for your food to move from your mouth to your anus is called the *transit time*. For most people, their transit time is anywhere from 15 to 48 hours, depending, in part, on the types of food they eat. For example, the transit time for fiber-rich food is much shorter than it is for meat. Some people just naturally have transit times that vary from slow to rapid.

The chomper

Digestion begins in the mouth and ends in the small intestine. The digestive process begins when you put food in your mouth and chew until it is soft and small enough to be swallowed. Swallowing moves the food down your esophagus and into your stomach.

The masher

The stomach is where the food we eat makes its first stop. The average stomach can hold 1 to 1½ quarts of food and liquid. Some stomachs can hold much more. The muscles in the lining of the stomach mix the food and liquid with digestive juices turning them into a thick liquid called chyme. Depending on the type of food you eat, this process can take anywhere from two to six hours. When the processing is complete, your stomach moves the chyme to its last stop in the upper GI track, the small intestine.

As you can see in Figures 3.1 and 3.5, the stomach is not below the belly button where children often think it is. The area around the belly button is closer to the transverse colon, which is where children frequently experience discomfort caused by constipation. This is why we teach children that what they may think is a "stomach ache" may actually be their body's way of telling them that they are constipated.

The extractor

The small intestine is where fats, starches and proteins are broken down into different acids and sugars and then absorbed into the bloodstream and transported throughout the body. Children are surprised to learn that the small intestine is approximately 20 feet long and 1 inch in diameter, like a piled up garden hose. Once our food is fully digested, the muscles of the small intestine push the left over liquid waste into the large intestine, or colon.

Figure 3.4 Small Intestine

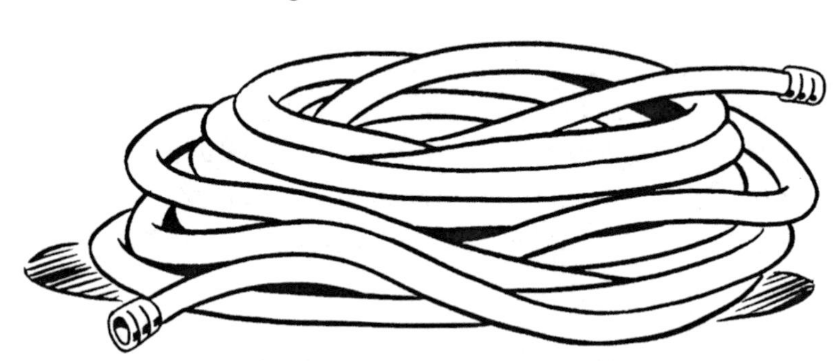

The poop factory

The large intestine, for the purpose of this discussion, is made up of the colon and the rectum. Technically, the rectum is the end section of the colon. The functions of the colon and the rectum are to absorb water and partially-digested food from the mostly liquid waste it receives from the small intestine and send the remaining waste through the anus and out of the body in the form of stool.

The colon is a tube which is approximately 5 feet long and 2 ½ to 3 inches in diameter. It is composed of five sections that become progressively narrower in diameter. Starting where the small intestine ends and moving from right to left, the sections are as follows:

- Ascending colon
- Transverse colon
- Descending colon
- Sigmoid colon
- Rectum

Figure 3.5 Large Intestine

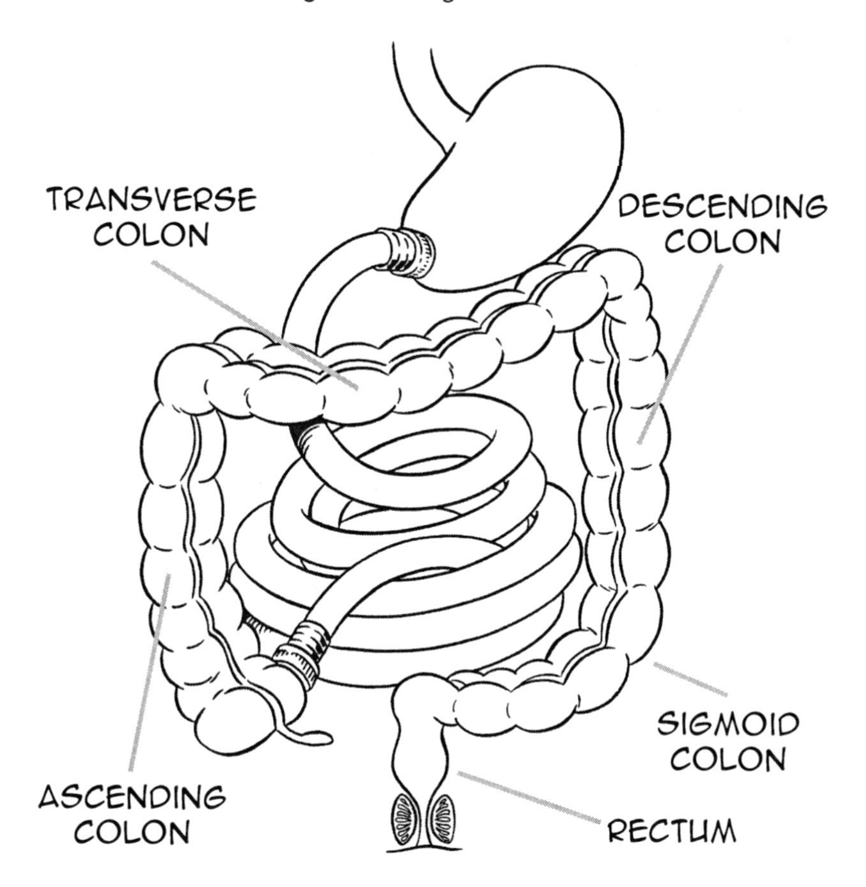

The poop collector

All sections of the colon are important, but the rectum plays an especially critical role. It is the final straight portion of the colon which serves as a temporary storage site for poop.

Stretches and urges

As the rectum fills with stool, stretch receptors in the walls of the rectum stimulate an urge to poop. If this initial feeling of readiness is not acted upon, stool is returned to the rectum or further back up to the sigmoid colon where more water is absorbed. When the rectum is full and the urge to poop cannot be ignored, a round muscle called the internal anal sphincter involuntarily opens, though only briefly (approximately ten seconds), allowing peristaltic waves to propel stool out of the rectum. Voluntary relaxation (opening) of another round muscle called the external anal sphincter allows stool to exit through the anus.

Chapter Notes

1. Seidel, E., Long, M.S., Cheshire, E. (2006). Crash Course: Gastrointestinal System. Philadelphia, PA: Elsevier, Inc.
2. National Digestive Diseases Information Clearinghouse (NDDIC). (2008, April). Your digestive system and how it works. (NIH Publication No. 08-2681). Retrieved 6/10/12 from http://digestive.niddk.nih.gov/ddiseases/pubs/yrdd/

Slowdown on the Poop Assembly Line

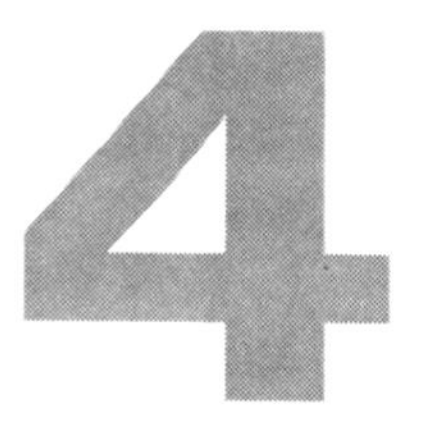

Occasional constipation

Occasional constipation is normal. For your child it means that stool is moving more slowly than usual through his or her large intestine. At one time or another, almost all children experience dry, hard stools that are difficult to pass. When constipation is mild, it may resolve on its own or require only minimal involvement on your part. In such cases it begins and ends fairly quickly, typically within one to two weeks.

Signs of a slowdown

- Fewer bowel movements per week than usual
- Stool is larger than usual
- Straining/pushing harder than usual
- Stool is dark brown with cracks/lumps on surface

Why it slows down

■ Raw materials

Your child's diet or changes in your child's diet can cause constipation. Babies sometimes get constipated when switched from breast milk to formula or from formula to whole cow's milk or from baby food to solid food. Some children get constipated while on family vacations due to dehydration, eating different foods, and changed meal times. Insufficient dietary fiber is one of the major causes of constipation. Fiber passes through the stomach and the large intestine largely undigested, especially insoluble fiber. In the large intestine, fiber absorbs water and makes the stool larger, softer, and easier to pass. (Read chapter 14 to learn more about fiber.) Insufficient fluids and fiber are major contributing factors to constipation in children.

■ Couch potatoes

Exercise is important because it directly affects the movement of stool. Our large intestine works better when we are active. Children (and adults) frequently feel the urge to poop either during exercise or shortly thereafter. Children who are physically active are less likely to become constipated than those who are not.

■ Hold it!

It is common for children to occasionally ignore or resist the urge to poop or pee. Children often "have to go" when there are no bathrooms close by. While riding in the car, how often have you told your young son or daughter to "hold it" until you can find a restroom? Elementary school teachers train students to, "wait until recess" or "until the bell rings." Children learn very quickly and surprisingly early in life that withholding poop or pee can make the urge go away. Fortunately, the occasional withholding of stool is normal and does not affect colonic functioning.

■ Tuning out

Some children become so engrossed in an activity, especially when playing electronic games, that they completely "tune out" or ignore what's going on around them, including the urge to poop. In fact, when asked, many children admit that they ignore the urge to poop. Addiction is a word that often comes to mind when parents talk about their child's demands for screen-time. While I know of no research to prove it, my impression is that the recent explosion in the variety of electronic devices with screens available to children has lead to a corresponding increase in the incidence of childhood constipation.

■ It's boring!

Toddlers and preschoolers sometimes resist sitting on the toilet when they begin toilet training because "it's not fun" and "it takes too long." Constipation can also be precipitated by the stress children experience when parents either begin toilet training too early or become impatient or upset because their children are not cooperating.

■ I don't feel good

Children who are ill with a fever, even for a brief period of time, will sometimes become constipated because of dehydration, inactivity, or both. Constipation is also an unwanted side effect of certain medications used to treat other conditions.

■ I'm afraid!

Some children avoid going to the bathroom or sitting on the toilet because they imagine that something bad will happen. These children are often described as "immature" or "sensitive." They may be afraid of "loud" flushing sounds, water splashing up on their bottoms, or falling into the toilet and being flushed away. Older children often begin to withhold stool when they start school and find that the bathrooms are bigger, noisier, messier, and less private than at home. Some children are fearful because of things they have seen in movies or on television.

> **A Doctor's Report**
>
> *A 3-year-old boy who had been constipated for six weeks was brought to my office. He had previously moved his bowels approximately once a day and had been toilet trained for at least six months. However, the frequency of bowel movements had decreased to approximately every four days and his stools were usually hard. He had initially complained of anal discomfort and refused to move his bowels. Eventually, he began to move his bowels but only infrequently and only while standing up and wearing a diaper. He adamantly refused to sit on the toilet and*

would ask for a diaper to be put on whenever he needed to move his bowels."

Results of my examination of the boy were normal. A rectal examination showed no stool because he had recently moved his bowels. Treatment with a mineral oil preparation resulted in improvement in the character of his stools and the return of his regular, daily bowel movements. However, he persisted in moving his bowels only while standing up and wearing a diaper. His mother believed his refusal to use the toilet was uncharacteristic of her son. Furthermore, he refused to divulge his reason for not wanting to sit on the toilet. Finally, he gave in to his mother's constant asking and told her that he had seen a television commercial advertisement in which a toilet bowel was portrayed as turning into a monster with the seat cover making a chomping movement. This image scared him from again sitting on the toilet; he feared that it "would get him." At present, efforts are directed at encouraging the patient, with much support and reassurances, to use the toilet. The family is having some success, although not consistently.[1]

■ Imaginary fears

Toilet or bathroom avoidance caused by imaginary fears may be particularly difficult for you as a parent to deal with because you may not be aware of your child's fears. All you know is that your child refuses to sit on the toilet or to go into the bathroom. You might naturally assume that your child is just being uncooperative. However, since young children find it difficult to describe or verbalize their fears, it may be months later, if ever, before you learn the real reason for your child's behavior.

■ It hurts!

Painful diaper rashes and anal fissures also cause children to withhold stool. If your child has uncomfortable or painful bowel movements, he or she may come to associate them with pain and begin to withhold stool whenever the urge is felt. Each time this happens, the stool is returned to the rectum where it becomes dryer, harder and even more difficult to pass.

Beware of withholding!

Prolonged withholding is the major cause of functional constipation in children. This is the reason why parents need to know right away if their child is constipated. Early intervention can prevent withholding or stop its progression before it gets out of your child's control.

Chapter Notes

1. Virgilio, P. R. (1990). A horrifying television commercial that led to constipation. *Pediatrics*, 85, 592–593.

Speeding Up the Poop Assembly Line

5

Treating occasional constipation

The key to preventing functional constipation is to treat occasional constipation early enough to avoid or minimize withholding. This means paying close attention to your child's bowel movements. You cannot assume that your child is having normal bowel movements just because he or she goes into the bathroom fairly regularly and you hear the toilet flush. At least once a week, I recommend that you observe your child pooping and inspect the poop. If you see one or more signs of occasional constipation as described in chapter 4, and the signs persist for more than a few days, initiate treatment with natural remedies. Laxatives are unnecessary for occasional constipation unless natural remedies are ineffective.

Poop food

Children in the United States consume about one half of the dietary fiber they need to produce healthy poop. The daily amount of fiber recommended for a child is 5 grams plus his age. For example, a 4-year-old child should consume 9 grams of fiber daily. As it is often difficult to get children to eat high-fiber foods, a synthetic substitute such as Benefiber is a good short-term substitute. See chapter 14 for more detailed information about fiber and fiber substitutes.

Let's go for a walk

Remember, our GI tract likes physical activity. Most children, especially preschool age children, get a sufficient amount of exercise. However, children who prefer sedentary activities, such as watching television or playing computer games, should be encouraged to be more active. You may need to foster your child's interest in activities that require more physical exertion, such as walking, jogging, bike riding, jump roping, or skate boarding. The best way to motivate your child to be more active is be active yourself. Participate along with your child and make it as enjoyable as possible for both of you.

Less moo

Dairy products do not always cause constipation, but the consumption of milk and cheese is so often associated with constipation that it makes sense to decrease, if not eliminate, milk and cheese from the diet, at least until your child is no longer constipated.

Check the label

Some medications can cause constipation. If your child is taking a medication such as an antibiotic for another condition, ask your healthcare provider or pharmacist if it causes constipation. If so, ask if a non-constipating alternative is available. If there is no alternative, change your child's diet by increasing fiber and decreasing milk and cheese. This should help relieve constipation more quickly once the medication is no longer needed.

Butt support

Make sure that your child has an age appropriate toilet seat and that his or her posture while pooping is conducive to moving stool. The seat should support your child's tailbone and the height of the seat should allow your child's feet to lie flat on the floor or on a stool. See chapter 12 for more detailed information about toilet seats and posture.

Eat first

Poop begins to move more quickly through the large intestine whenever we eat, which is why we often feel the urge to poop during meals or shortly thereafter. The physiological process responsible for this is called the gastrocolic reflex (see chapter 3). Children (and adults) often ignore urgency after eating because they are too busy. Encouraging your child to sit on the toilet shortly after eating will increase the likelihood of your child having a bowel movement.

Within a week or two, the majority of children who develop occasional constipation respond positively to one or more of the natural remedies and their poop returns to normal. Their bowel movements are more frequent, their poop is again shaped more like a banana than a log, the edges of their poop are smooth not cracked and lumpy, and the poop's color is light brown not dark brown.

If your child is still constipated after a week or two, or you see early warning signs of functional constipation, consider starting your child on a laxative.

Warning signs of functional constipation

- Bowel movements "hurt"
- Four or fewer bowel movements a week
- Lower abdominal tummy aches
- Large diameter stools that block the toilet

Persistent, discomfort or pain during bowel movements can quickly lead to habitual withholding. The only way to prevent habitual withholding and functional constipation is to keep your child's poop very soft for as long as necessary. If natural remedies do no work, laxatives are necessary.

The misunderstood laxative

Parents who are unfamiliar with laxatives are understandably concerned about giving them to their children. However, water retention laxatives are frequently recommended for children for the relief of occasional constipation that does not respond to natural remedies. Water retention laxatives hold or draw water into the large intestine to keep stool moist and soft. In a sense, they act like fiber but more efficaciously.

Polyethylene glycol 3350 (PEG) is the most commonly recommended water retention laxative for children. It is available in your local pharmacy under a number of different brand names. A prescription is not required.

Is it safe?

Although not approved by the Food and Drug Administration specifically for use in children, polyethylene glycol (PEG) is considered by many pediatric healthcare providers to be the "gold standard" laxative for children. It is a tasteless, odorless powder that is mixed in 6-8 ounces of water or some other liquid such as fruit juice.

How much?

Some children are more sensitive than others to polyethylene glycol laxative products. Therefore, the standard dose recommended on the container may not be enough or may be too much. The standard dose may not soften your child's poop, or it may make the poop too loose or watery. If this happens, it is okay to give more or less than the recommended dose. See chapter 10 for more information about oral laxatives.

When to stop

DO NOT STOP THE LAXATIVE TOO SOON. The goal for your child is at least three months of daily soft poops with no recurrence of withholding and/or any of the warning signs of functional constipation. Once your child achieves this goal, decrease the laxative by one-half for seven days and then discontinue the laxative altogether. If withholding or any of the early warning signs of functional constipation reoccur, go back to the earlier dose but this time wait four weeks before trying to lower the dose a second time.

Stopping Laxatives Too Soon

My son Elijah had his first experience with constipation when he was about 3 years old. We encouraged him to drink more juice and we added more fiber to his diet but that did not stop the screaming and bottom clenching each time he had a bowel movement. I talked to my pediatrician who recommended that I give Elijah a laxative. I was so desperate at that point that I was willing to give it a try. He told us to keep using it until Elijah wasn't constipated anymore. It didn't take long for Elijah to get some relief, and us, too. It's hard as a parent to watch your child be in pain and not know what to do to help him. Just as the doctor ordered, we stopped giving Elijah the laxative as soon as his bowel movements softened and his pain went away. We then assumed that if we just put him on a high fiber diet he would be okay.

However, not long after we stopped the laxative, Elijah again became afraid that his bowel movements would hurt and he began to resist sitting on the toilet to poop. So, once again, he became constipated. Coincidentally, we were away from home on vacation when this happened, where I happened to meet Dr. DuHamel ("Dr. Tom") who gave us some helpful advice. He advised me to put Elijah back on the laxative and to keep him on it for at least three months. He also suggested that we try massaging Elijah's tummy while he was sitting on the toilet and that we have him sit on the toilet a little longer than we had before. We were so thankful that we got that advice when we did!

> *It didn't happen overnight, but once Elijah was able to relax and he knew that it wasn't going to hurt every time he went to the bathroom, he began to go more regularly.* • **Sarah H.**

If withholding or any other early warning signs reoccur following your second attempt at stopping the laxative, consult with your child's healthcare provider immediately.

Poop Assembly Line Shutdown

Functional constipation

All of us, children and adults alike, withhold bowel movements almost every day, either because there is no bathroom close by or because the timing is inconvenient. Severely constipated children withhold in order to avoid uncomfortable or painful bowel movements.

Withholding

Children who experience pain or discomfort when pooping quickly learn that the pain or discomfort can be avoided by simply contracting the muscle (sphincter) around their anus whenever they feel the need to poop. Withholding begins as a voluntary response, but if the painful or uncomfortable bowel movements continue, withholding can become involuntary. This means that the anal muscle "closes" automatically whenever the rectum contracts. Withholding is no longer a conscious decision. It has become a habit.

Exactly how long it takes for withholding to become a habit varies with age and temperament. Some infants and children begin to withhold involuntarily after just one uncomfortable bowel movement whereas others are able to tolerate a number of uncomfortable bowel movements before becoming habitual withholders. The difference between the two groups is most likely related to the degree of discomfort or pain they experience.

The more intense the discomfort the more quickly withholding becomes involuntary.

Two types of withholding

Clinical experience suggests that there are two types of withholding: complete and incomplete.

1. *Complete withholding* is when the anal muscle closes tightly each time the rectum contracts. This prevents any poop from passing.
2. *Incomplete withholding* is when the anal muscle does not close completely, which allows some but not the entire amount of poop in the rectum to pass.

Behavioral signs of withholding

If your child is withholding, you are likely to observe one or more of the following behaviors.

- Clenching/squeezing of the buttocks
- Extending or stiffening the body
- Crossing legs/ankles
- Excessive rocking or fidgeting
- Squatting with heel in crack of buttocks

Figure 6.1
Withholding Postures

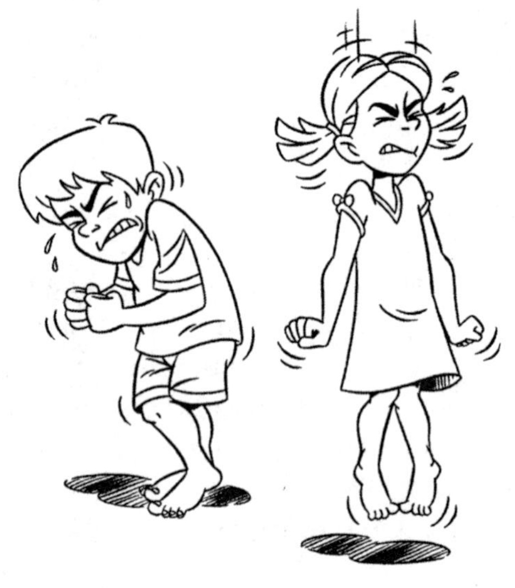

Withholding and the rectum

The rectum stretches (distends) in order to accommodate both the old (retained) poop and the new poop entering from higher up in the colon. If the duration of stretching is brief, the rectum will soon shrink back to its normal size. However, if the rectum is stretched for an extended period of time, it becomes enlarged and may take months or even years to recover.

Think of the rectum as a muscle with a hole in the middle. Like other hollow organs that become enlarged, such as the uterus during pregnancy, an enlarged rectum will begin to have frequent contractions. As the rectum repeatedly stretches and contracts, its walls become thicker and stronger. A normally functioning rectum is sensitive to increased amounts of poop and will trigger accurate and consistent feelings of urgency as it fills. An enlarged (stronger) rectum loses its sensitivity, leaving your child unaware that his rectum is filling and that he will soon need to poop.

Figure 6.2 Normal and Enlarged Rectum

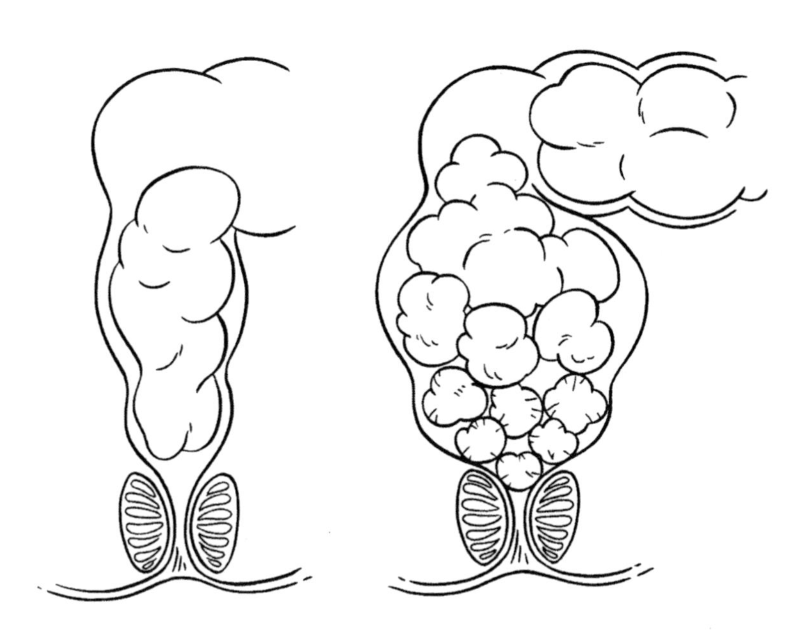

Accidental incontinence

If withholding is complete, the poop retained in the rectum will dry fairly quickly forming a dry, hard mass. Soft, moist poop from above the rectum works its way around the mass and leaks out into your child's underwear. Initial incontinence may be a watery poop that parents sometimes confuse with diarrhea. But as withholding continues and poop continues to accumulate, incontinence progresses from liquid, to streaks or smears and then to full bowel movements.

When withholding is incomplete, it may take months or years for a child's rectum to stretch to the point where it begins to contract abnormally and cause incontinence. With incomplete withholding, "accidents" are not watery and, regardless of size, are more apt to be soft than hard. Because the child's poop is mostly soft and he poops frequently, parents and healthcare providers often do not realize that the child is constipated.

Stool incontinence is one of the most frustrating and annoying constipation-related behaviors parents have to deal with. It is what leads them and their healthcare providers to conclude that these children have serious emotional problems or that they are developmentally delayed. Some children who are incontinent do have emotional or developmental problems, but the vast majority does not. Some children who are incontinent are strong-willed and defiant but no more so than other children of their age.[1]

Physical signs of rectal stretching

Abdominal protrusion

A common telltale sign of prolonged rectal distention is lower abdominal protrusion in the area just below a child's belly button where the lateral section of the colon is located.

Figure 6.3 Abdominal Protrusion

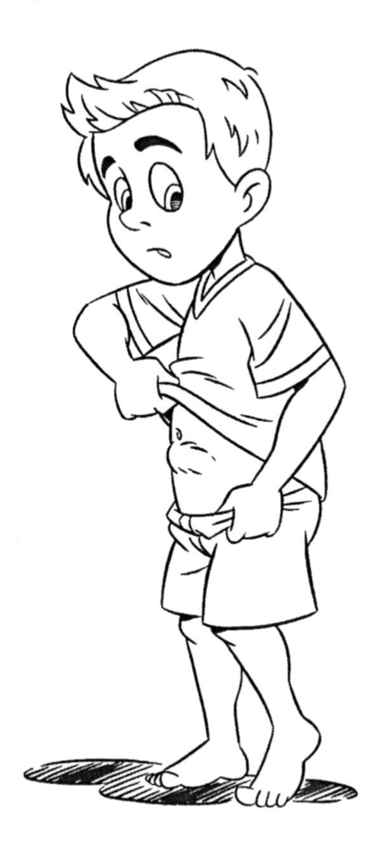

Stomach aches, nausea, and vomiting

Each child responds differently to having an enlarged rectum. Responses vary with a child's age, temperament, tolerance for pain, and other medical conditions. Some children experience lower abdominal pain or cramps, which they describe as stomach or "tummy" aches. Other children experience heartburn. Decreased appetite is common. This is not surprising since we know that even minimal rectal distention delays the passage of a meal through the stomach. Some children feel so "full" that they become nauseous and may even vomit when presented with more food.

Wetting accidents

Nighttime wetting or daytime dripping and leaking are frequently due to a distended rectum. In Figure 6.4, note how close the rectum is to the urinary bladder. If one or both of these organs are full they can easily press up against one another, increasing the chance of accidental wetting. This is especially true for children who wait until the last second to urinate.

Figure 6.4 Bladder/Rectum Proximity

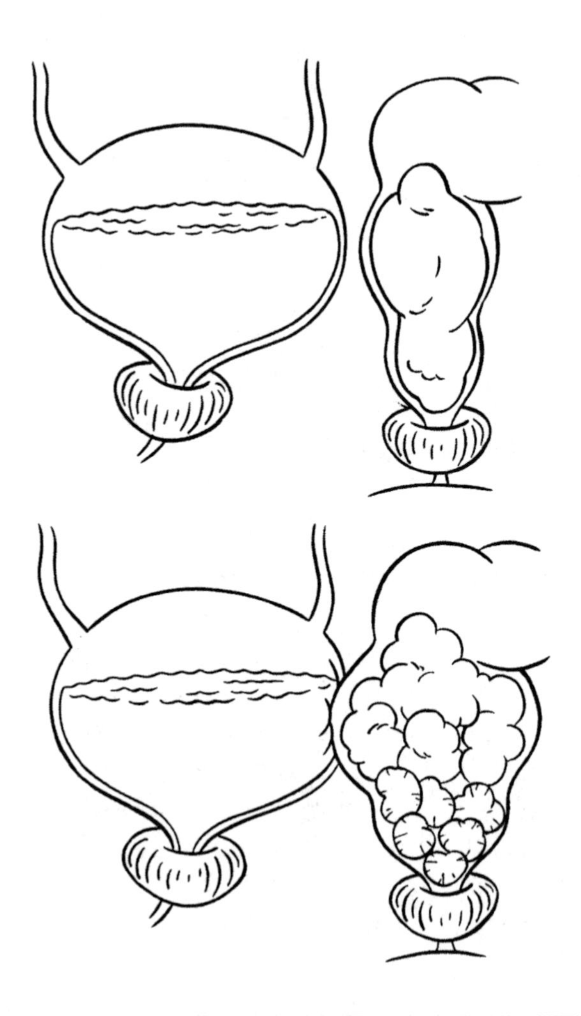

Emotional and behavioral signs of rectal stretching

Mood changes

Lethargy, irritability and mood changes that are otherwise unexplainable may be due to an enlarged rectum. For example, an 11-year-old boy was referred because of concerns about recurring episodes of extreme lethargy and disinterest in activities he typically enjoyed. His parents wanted to know if he was depressed. Upon evaluation, it was learned that this young man's bowel movements were routinely about ten days apart and that his lethargy and disinterest disappeared almost immediately after a large bowel movement, only to gradually increase again until his next bowel movement. This boy's parents thought the ten-day span was just their son's "normal bowel pattern." They neither realized that he was constipated nor that functional constipation can impact a child's mood and behavior.

Hiding soiled underwear

Some children resist or refuse removing their soiled underwear while others will secretly remove their soiled underwear and then hide them. It is not clear why children do this, especially when most of them have been told many times that they will not be punished for having an accident, but that they will be punished for hiding their soiled underwear.

Denial

Parents are baffled by children who deny having had an accident even though everyone around them can smell it. When questioned, these children will say, "I don't smell poop, and I don't feel it on my bottom." Hearing this upsets parents. If everyone else can smell it, surely their children can smell it. The children must be lying. Or are they?

It is possible that these children are telling the truth. Just as there are heavy smokers who are unable to smell smoke in their clothing, there are severely constipated children who are unable to smell poop in their underwear. These children are desensitized to the smell of poop just like long-term smokers are desensitized to the smell of smoke. It might also be true that these children do not feel poop on their skin. As stool passes through the anal opening, it is at body temperature and, therefore, less likely to be noticed.

Why they hide and deny

Although no one to my knowledge has researched this question, I have observed that many children who hide and deny have struggled with this problem for a long time with little or no success. In their minds, they have done everything their parents and their doctors have told them to do, yet they still have accidents and their parents still get upset. They are discouraged and they just want their "poop problem" to go away. For them, hiding and denying is the sort of "out of sight, out of mind" thinking that we all engage in from time to time when faced with a difficult problem. If I am overweight but never weigh myself, it is easier for me to think that I don't have a weight problem. Similarly, for these children, if they deny or hide their accidents it is easier for them to think that they do not have a poop problem.

Chapter Notes

1. Blum, N. J., Taubman, B., & Osborne, M. L. (1997). Behavioral characteristics of children with stool toileting refusal. *Pediatrics*, 99, 50–53.

Put On Your Work Clothes

7

Treatment is hard work

Patience pays off

If your child needs treatment for functional constipation, be prepared for what lies ahead. It is not going to be easy for you, your child, or your family. Helping a child with functional constipation requires more patience than you can imagine. Treatment can last for months or years depending on initial severity. The good news is that with comprehensive care, functional constipation can be dramatically improved.[1]

Coping with uncertainty

Parents must be able to cope with uncertainty. Lower abdominal x-rays tell us how much stool is in the rectum and whether the rectum appears to be enlarged. However, x-rays do not give us a metric by which we can tell how much larger a child's rectum is relative to normal. In fact, we don't even know what normal means with regard to the size of a child's rectum because it is quite likely that rectal size varies from one child to another. We know that retained stool causes the rectum to stretch, but we have no way of measuring exactly how much it has stretched. We give laxatives to keep stool soft so that the rectum can shrink, yet we also have no way of knowing when it begins to shrink or how much shrinkage has occurred at any point during the course of treatment.

The only changes we can accurately verify and quantify are symptom changes such as the frequency and consistency of bowel movements. Adding more uncertainty is the fact that symptom changes can be caused by factors unrelated to treatment, such as a change in diet or illness.

Laxative choices

Another uncertainty is which laxative to choose. A laxative that works for one child may not work for another. This is especially true for stimulant laxatives. How much laxative a child needs is unclear. Dosing changes, based on symptoms such as stool consistency at the beginning and during the course of treatment, are often necessary. Laxative decisions are further complicated by whether or not your child will agree to take a particular laxative because of how it tastes or smells.

Your child's treatment will consume a lot of your time and energy. You will need to make sure that the right amount of laxative is taken every day and that your child sits on the toilet after meals. In most cases, you also will need to be in the bathroom to help focus your child on the reason for being there and to ensure that "pushing" is done properly. You will need to watch for withholding or accidents and collect data regarding bowel movements and laxative use.

No matter how patient and understanding you are, it is inevitable that there will be times when you feel angry and resentful. "He should take more responsibility for his bowel movements!" "I should not have to remind her all the time!" These thoughts and feelings are normal and healthy under the circumstances. Just do the best you can. Remember, your child wants this problem to go away just as much as you do.

Figure 7.1 Mom at Work

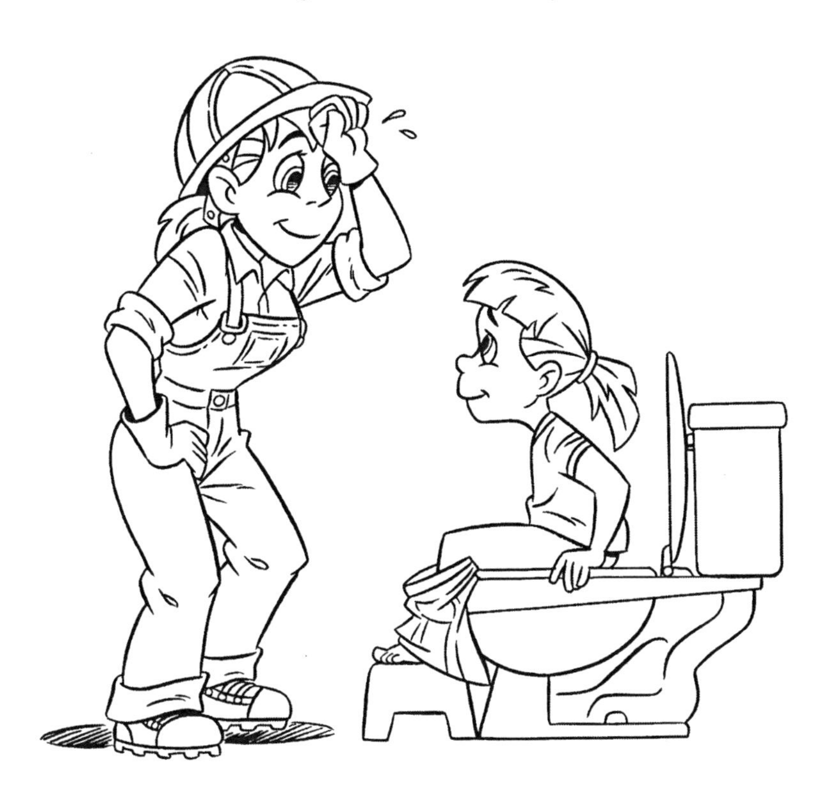

Chapter Notes

1. Loening-Baucke, V. (2002). Functional fecal retention in childhood. *Practical Gastroenterology*, 25, 213–21.

Restarting The Poop Assembly Line

8

How to treat functional constipation

Part 1 - Treating Fear

To stop withholding and allow the rectum to begin its lengthy recovery, we must first decrease your child's underlying fear. Parents frequently ask why their child continues to withhold even when bowel movements do not hurt. The answer is that these children have become conditioned to expect pain if they relax their poop muscle.

Irrational fear

Continuing to fear pain in the absence of pain seems irrational. Although there was a reason to be afraid in the past, that reason no longer exists. Irrational fears or phobias, such as fear of bees following a bee sting, can persist for a long time, even when the original stimulus does not recur. Such fears require treatment with *exposure therapy.*

Exposure therapy

In exposure therapy, phobic fears are neutralized by gradually and repeatedly exposing people to the object or situation that evokes their fear. A severely constipated child's fear of pain decreases little by little each time he passes stool and does not experience pain. If you put a drop of red food coloring into a small glass of water, the water turns a deep red. But if you put that same amount of food coloring into a gallon of water, the color of the water may not change at all. The red color (fear) gradually decreases as the amount of water (number of painless bowel movements) increases.

Figure 8.1 Decreasing Fear

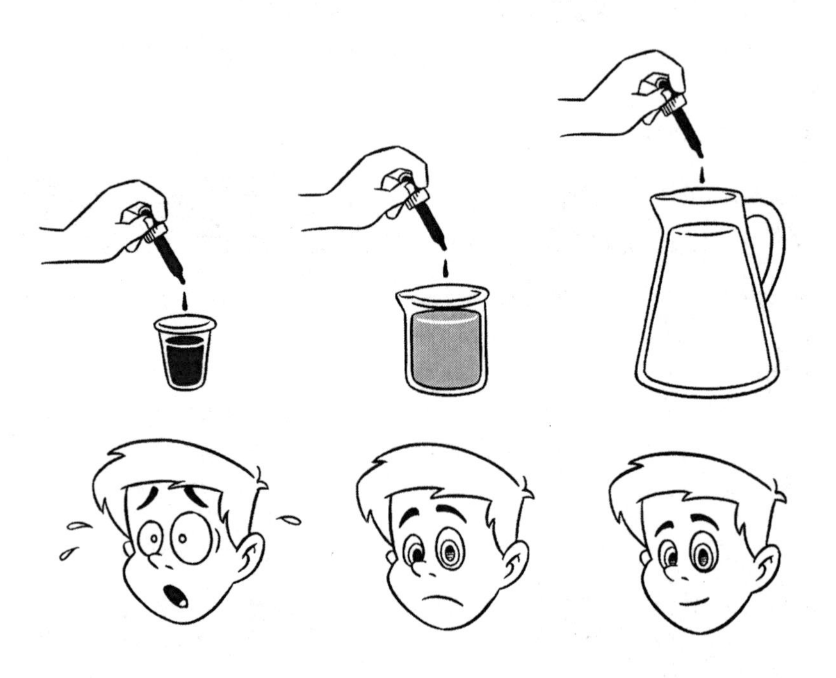

The number of pain-free bowel movements required to neutralize or extinguish the fear of pain varies from child to child depending on various factors such as the age at which constipation began and the child's current level of maturity and cooperation. Regardless of these individual differences, however, the number of painless bowel movements required is always going to be large, which is why the treatment of functional constipation takes so long and why incentives are so essential (see chapter 13).

Irrational fear expands

Irrational fears often generalize or expand. Just as children withhold poop in order to avoid pain, they sometimes refuse to sit on the toilet or go into the bathroom for the same reason. Just sitting on the toilet or being in the bathroom for the purpose of pooping evokes the fear of pain.

Pooping in other places

No matter where they are, children may all of a sudden become quiet, look as though they are "lost in thought," poop in their underwear and then continue on like nothing happened. Some children will move to another room or hide behind a couch or chair to poop while others will poop while engaged in a solitary activity such as playing with Legos.

Pooping in Pull-ups

Some children avoid the toilet and the bathroom by refusing to poop unless they are wearing a diaper or a Pull-up. A small percentage of these children have never had a bowel movement sitting on the toilet. A larger percentage have had bowel movements on the toilet in the past but stopped once they experienced pain. Some parents put their children back into diapers or Pull-ups as a way of helping them relax to poop. Other parents do it as a way of managing the messiness of poop accidents.

Whatever the reason, be cautious about allowing a child to regress by putting him back into diapers or Pull-ups. Although there are definitely good reasons to do so, be aware that children will sometimes become dependent on diapers or Pull-ups for peeing as well as for pooping which can make it even harder to get them back to using the toilet.

Fear is always present

"If my child is afraid to poop in the toilet or in the bathroom, why isn't he afraid to poop in other rooms in the house?" Good question. Remember that your child's fear is irrational, like a phobia. The fear is always present no matter where he goes, but it is not as strong outside the bathroom as it is inside the bathroom. As with a spider phobia, the fear is greatest in the presence of a spider but less if you only see a picture of a spider.

It is easier for your child to relax his poop muscle if he is away from the toilet and the bathroom. He can more easily distract himself from the fear of pain by playing quietly in his room or by playing outside. By moving to another room or by hiding, he can also avoid any additional stress that you might cause by getting upset or by telling him to poop in the bathroom.

The good news is that most of these children have no problem using the bathroom for other reasons such as bathing or brushing teeth. Most of them will also use the toilet to urinate, even those who need diapers or Pull-ups to poop.

Parental participation

When your child is afraid to do something such as going to the dentist, you do not make him go alone. You know that he is comforted by your presence and that his dental appointment will be more successful if you are there with him. The same is true for a child with functional constipation. Even if your child does not say he is afraid or does not appear to be afraid, he *is* afraid. This is just one reason why it is so important for you to be an active participant in all aspects of your child's treatment, especially whenever he sits on the toilet.

Part 2 - Six-Step Program

Once withholding stops and excess poop is no longer retained, the rectum slowly shrinks back to its normal size. Incontinence decreases as the rectum shrinks and regains its ability to signal bowel urgency. The time required to stop withholding and for the rectum to shrink to its normal size differs from one child to another. Generally, the longer a child has been constipated the longer it takes for both. The time required to stop withholding ranges from three to six months. It can take another three months to a year or longer for the rectum to return to its normal size.

For a child to be able to stop withholding, he or she must be able to pass large quantities of stool every day without pain or discomfort. For this to happen, the stool must be very soft. Laxatives are almost always necessary.

STEP 1. Educate the family

Education is the critical first step to successful treatment. To complete this step:

1. Make an appointment with your pediatric healthcare provider.
2. Educate yourself, your child, and other family members about constipation.
3. Begin collecting data regarding the frequency of bowel movements and the consistency of your child's poop.

Meet with your healthcare provider

Your healthcare provider will ask you questions about your child's constipation. Show your provider the data you have recorded on the "Weekly Laxative and Stool Record" (see Appendix). Your child's medical history and a routine physical examination are usually all that is necessary for your provider to make a diagnosis of functional constipation. Your healthcare provider will first explain the treatment plan, starting with the initial cleanout, and then schedule a follow-up office visit or telephone call to determine whether a second cleanout will be needed.

Educate yourself and your child

If you read this entire book, you will learn all you need to know about functional constipation. Chapter 9 has sample instructions for educating your child about how our bodies process food and waste, what happens when we become constipated, and how laxatives work. If you have any questions, be sure to ask your healthcare provider during your initial or follow-up appointments.

Begin data collection

Collecting information about your child's elimination on a daily basis is important for a number of reasons. It will help you and your healthcare provider determine whether the initial cleanout was sufficient or whether another cleanout should be done. Moreover, during the long course of treatment, the "Weekly Laxative and Stool Record" will help you keep track of important information. For example, is your child having one or more poops a day? Is the poop mostly soft, or is it too hard or too loose? Laxative changes or dose adjustments should be based not on only one or two days' worth of data but on trends seen in data collected over a number of weeks. Recording this data every day for weeks and months is tedious but critical for treatment success.

STEP 2. Empty the rectum

Cleaning out the rectum takes 1–4 days. Completing this step involves:

1. Rapid removal of backed up dry/hard poop from the large intestine.
2. Use of high doses of mineral oil, oral laxatives, or a rectal laxative.
3. Collecting data about your child's poops.

How much excess poop?

Prior to the start of Step 2 your child's healthcare provider may determine the extent of your child's constipation by inserting a finger into your child's rectum (digital exam), pressing on your child's lower abdomen (palpation), or x-ray studies. Excess poop may be mostly in the rectum, or it may also be higher up in the sigmoid, transverse and ascending sections of the colon. (See Figure 3.5.) The complete removal of large quantities of retained poop may require more than one cleanout.

Laxative choices and dosages

Cleanouts are frequently done with high doses of a lubricant laxative such as mineral oil and/or high doses of polyethylene glycol (PEG). Cleanouts can take up to four days and are usually done over a weekend when parents are not working and children are not in daycare or school. The higher than usual doses necessary for cleanouts often make poop so loose that it leaks out uncontrollably into a child's diaper or underwear.

Some healthcare providers prefer to use a rectally administered laxative for cleanouts. An enema or a suppository removes excess poop more quickly and predictably than oral laxatives; however, most children resist them and parents are generally uneasy about administering them. Nevertheless, used properly, rectal laxatives are a viable alternative to oral laxatives and should be considered. You can learn more about rectal laxatives and how to administer them in chapter 11.

Is it cleaned out?

After the initial cleanout it is sometimes difficult to know if all or most of the retained poop has been removed. Success is determined by the amount of poop that is passed but this is often hard to quantify because the poop is likely to be very soft or mushy. Your healthcare provider may want to see your child again to make a determination either by palpation or by a second x-ray before moving on to the next step in the treatment plan.

STEP 3. End withholding

Ending withholding takes 3 to 6 months. Completing this step requires the following:

1. Find the most efficacious laxative(s) and dosage.
2. Establish a daily routine of sitting and pushing.
3. Use incentives to motivate and reinforce cooperation.
4. Continue your data collection.

The goal of Step 3 is to find the combination of laxatives and behavioral strategies that will enable your child to consistently push out one or two soft large bowel movements every day with no signs of withholding. Rectal normalization (Step 4) cannot begin until withholding stops.

Step 3 is the phase of treatment during which your child's association of pain with urgency is gradually extinguished together with his related habit of withholding. For many families this is the most confusing and frustrating phase of treatment. Keep in mind that your child is probably just as confused and discouraged as you are. Try to be patient. Your child feels trapped by his constipation just as much as you do.

Dosage changes

Your child's healthcare provider may decide to use a lower dose of the same laxative(s) used for the cleanout or to use a different laxative. Not one laxative or one dose of a laxative works for all children. Finding the most efficacious laxative and the best dose of that laxative is often a process of trial and error which, at times, can cause a child's stools to become either too hard or too soft. You will find more information about laxatives and how to administer them in chapter 10.

During this trial and error process it is not uncommon for a child to again become constipated or incontinent.

Warning! Too much of a laxative can cause stool incontinence. This incontinence is due to medication, not to constipation. Increasing the dose of laxatives will only make the incontinence worse.

Sitting and pushing schedule

Sitting and pushing one to three times a day is necessary in order to reach the goal of passing a large amount of poop every day. Detailed information about sitting schedules and about teaching a child to push correctly can be found in chapter 12.

Incentives for cooperation

There are many reasons why children do not cooperate with treatment. Some resist, some refuse, while others simply deny that there is a problem. Enlisting your child's cooperation requires the use of positive incentives. Punishment or the threat of punishment does not work and can be counterproductive. You will learn more about positive and negative incentives in chapter 13.

STEP 4. Shrink the Rectum

Shrinking the rectum can take three to twelve months or longer. This step requires that you:

1. Continue with Step 3.
2. Watch for withholding.
3. Make laxative dose adjustments.
4. Watch for the decrease/stopping of stool incontinence.
5. Continue data collection.

This is the phase of treatment when we expect the rectum to regain its normal muscle tone, elasticity and sensitivity. Unfortunately, it is impossible to determine when or whether the rectum has fully recovered. We assume that full recovery takes many months following the cessation of withholding because withholding often recurs when healthcare providers discontinue laxatives prematurely.

Dosage adjustments

Dosage adjustments during Step 4 should be based on changes in frequency, quantity, and consistency of bowel movements. Do not make adjustments unnecessarily or prematurely that might cause withholding or increased incontinence. If adjustments are needed, they are usually only minor adjustments such as an increase or decrease by 1 or ½ teaspoon. For this reason, I strongly recommend using measuring spoons with powdered laxatives, especially when trying to estimate less than a "one cap" dose. For reference, when dosing a PEG laxative, a cap (17 grams) is approximately 5 level teaspoons.

For example, if a child has two or more days without a bowel movement in a one-week period, or when the stool tends to be darker colored or lumpier than usual, I often recommend that the water retention laxative be increased by a small amount—just long enough to get the frequency and consistency of poop back to normal.

STEP 5. Withdraw laxatives

Withdrawing laxative takes 1-3 months or more. During this step you need to:

1. Determine when to start withdrawal.
2. Withdraw stimulant laxatives first.
3. Lower doses very gradually (e.g. by ½ tsp at a time).
4. Wait 4–5 days between reductions to assess effect.
5. Continue data collection.

WARNING! Do not stop laxatives abruptly. Constipation, withholding, and rectal stretching can reoccur quickly.

When to begin withdrawal

Since there is no way of knowing if or when the rectum has shrunk to its normal size, healthcare providers rely on past experience to decide when to begin the process of weaning a child from laxatives. The answer to this question is typically based on the amount of time required to stop withholding. If it took only 1 to 2 months to stop withholding, the withdrawal process can begin after 3 to 6 months of daily, medium to large, mostly banana shaped poops on the toilet. However, if it took longer than three months to stop the withholding, do not begin withdrawing laxatives until the child has passed normal poops without accidents for 7 to 12 months.

Lower doses gradually—stimulants first

Laxative doses should be reduced gradually, starting with stimulant laxatives, to slowly increase the firmness of poop retained in the rectum before it is released into the anal canal. Over time, the anal canal and the poop muscle have become accustomed to very soft, moist stool and need time to readjust to a more compact, heavier stool.

Wait 4 to 5 days

If the poop becomes drier and more compact too quickly, either because the dose was lowered too quickly or because there was too little time between dose reductions, the anal canal and the poop muscle may not have time to adjust. This could cause withholding and lead to even drier stools and a decrease in the frequency of bowel movements. If you see any of these signs of constipation, increase the dose back to its previous level and be sure to wait at least 4 to 5 days before attempting to lower it a second time. If you see signs of constipation on the second attempt, return to the previous level but this time wait at least a month before making another attempt, and so on.

STEP 6. Remain vigilant

Even after withholding has stopped and laxatives are tapered down or discontinued, you must still remain vigilant for at least another 6-12 months.

1. Assume that constipation will reoccur.
2. Encourage fiber-rich foods, liquids and exercise.
3. Monitor for changes in bowel movement frequency and consistency.

If it comes back

At the first sign of constipation, put your child back on the same dose of the laxative(s) he received at either the beginning or end of Step 5.

If it does not come back, congratulations! Give your child a hug and yourself a pat on the back. You both deserve it.

The ABC's of Constipation

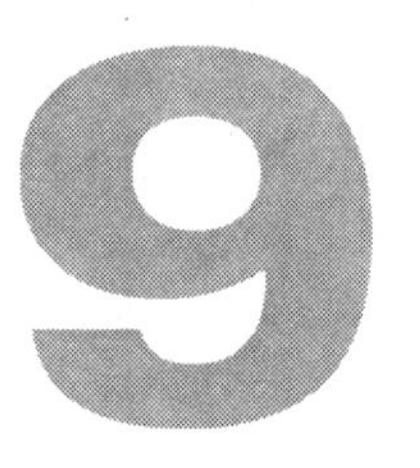

Educating children

Experts in the area of functional constipation (encopresis) all agree that the first step in treatment is for people to learn the facts about constipation. Acquiring this information has been referred to as the "demystification" of functional constipation. Knowledge about constipation is just as important for children as it is for parents. Like adults, children who are knowledgeable about constipation are more likely to be active participants in their treatment. For example, if children know that pain or discomfort in the lower abdomen might signal the need to poop, they may be more likely to sit on the toilet when they have a "tummy ache."

Repetition and learning

You cannot assume that your child will understand or remember what you have said about poop problems after only one or two explanations. Moreover, a 3- or 4-year-old child will not understand and retain as much information as a 5- or 6-year-old child, and so on. Parents, like all good teachers, should teach to the age and maturity level of their students.

What children need to learn

Children are naturally interested in their bodies' processes and by-products. Learning together about the ins and outs of poop can help you and your child become partners in the treatment plan. Topics to cover include:

- How our bodies make poop
- How our bodies tell us to poop
- Why poop gets hard and hurts
- Why we have poop "accidents"
- How poop medicine works

Visual aids and narratives

When it comes to poop, a picture *is* worth a thousand words. This is especially true when teaching children. The visual aid I recommend is an illustration showing the gastrointestinal tract from top to bottom. The key to effective teaching is to get and hold the learner's attention. A good visual aid helps capture a child's attention, but holding a child's attention requires an interesting and age-appropriate narrative and an entertaining narrator.

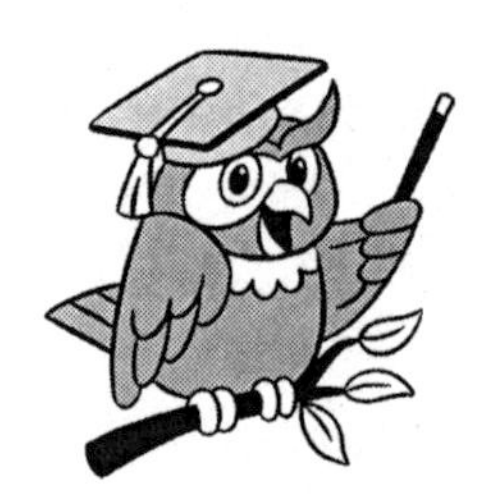

Narratives for children

The following is a generic version of the narrative I use, either in whole or in part, with more or less detail, depending upon the child's age and level of maturity. I show the drawing in Figure 9.1 and point out specific anatomy as I go. Each time I refer to one of the organs along the GI tract, I include two names, one for younger children and one for older children. Some children enjoy hearing both names. Take your pick and have fun!

Figure 9.1. GI Tract for Children

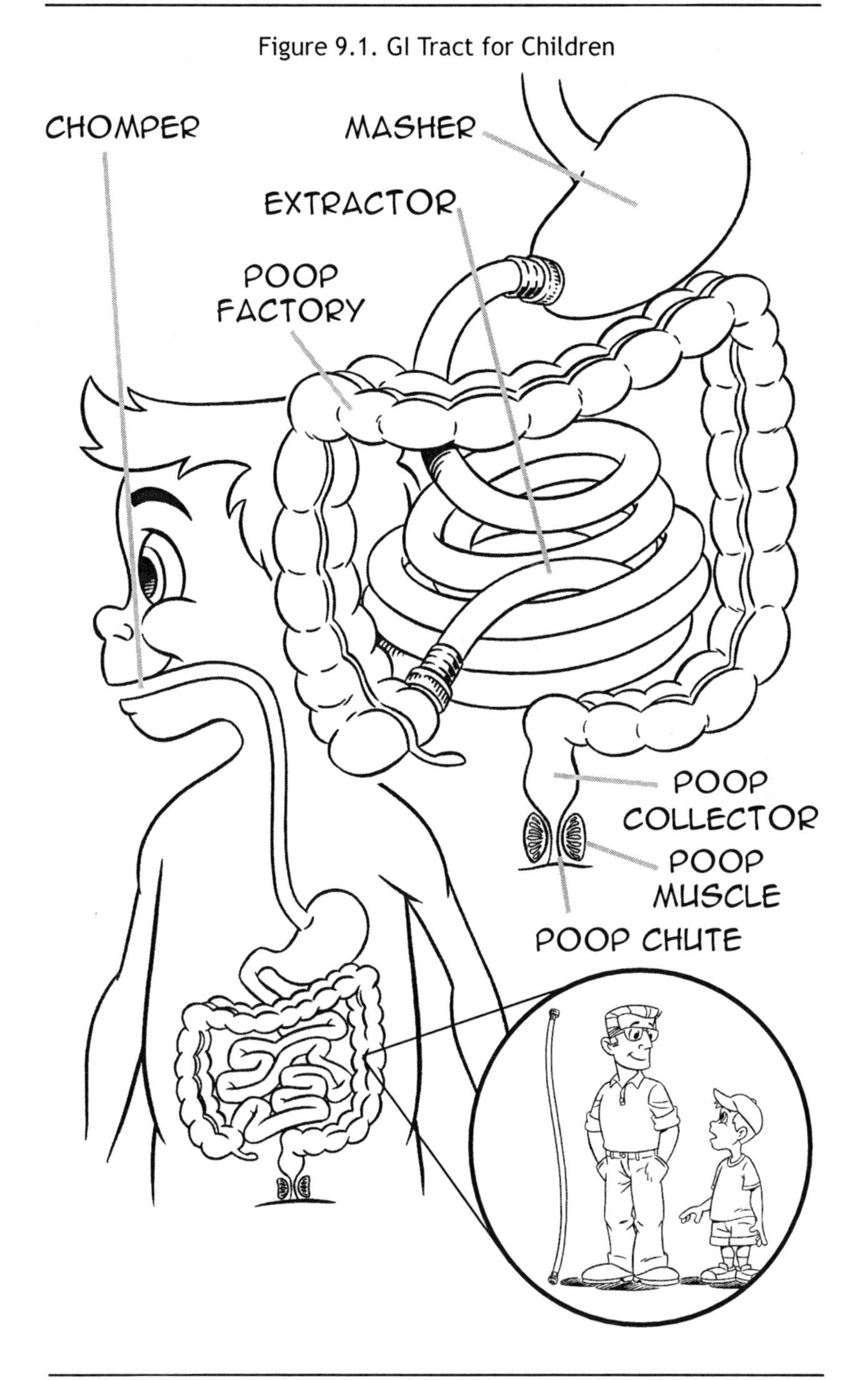

1. How your body makes poop

Explaining digestion

Julie, do you know how your body makes poop?	It begins when you put food in your chomper (mouth) and chew. Then, when you swallow, your food goes down a tube called the esophagus into your food masher (stomach).
Do you know what the masher (stomach) does?"	It turns food into something that looks like oatmeal. This is called digestion and the "oatmeal" is chyme.
Can you point to where your masher (stomach) is located in your body? Guess what? It's not down there. It's up here.	*If she points to the area below her belly button,* correct her by pointing out that it is in the upper left quadrant of her chest, above her belly button. When your masher (stomach) is done with your food, it goes through another tube into your extractor (small intestine). Your extractor (small intestine) looks sort of like a garden hose that is all curled up on itself.
Do you have a garden hose at home? Have your parents ever left it curled up in a pile on the ground?	That's what your extractor (small intestine) looks like.
Guess what happens to the "oatmeal" (chyme) when it goes into your extractor (small intestine)?	This is where your body takes out everything it needs to keep you healthy. Imagine that there are millions of little straws inside the walls of the extractor (small intestine) that suck out all of the vitamins and minerals you need to be strong and smart and to run fast.

	What's left over after your extractor (small intestine) takes out all the good things is called waste. The waste is then sent to your poop factory (large intestine) where your body turns it into poop (stool).
Explaining how stool is made	
Did you know that your poop factory (large intestine) is about six feet long?	That's about as tall as your dad! It starts on the lower right side of your body, comes up a bit and then crosses under your belly button. On your left side it goes down and then it goes around to the back side of your body to where your poop comes out. I call this the "poop chute" because it's where your poop comes out of your body.
Now, let's talk about how the poop factory (large intestine) works. Do you have chores?	Your poop factory (large intestine) has two chores (jobs) to do. One of the poop factory's (large intestine's) jobs is to take water out of your poop. Its other job is to keep your poop moving quickly so that it doesn't take out too much water, because if it takes out too much water, your poop will get dry and hard and it could hurt you when it comes out your poop chute.
What happens if you don't do your chores? Your parents are unhappy, right?	Well, if the poop factory (large intestine) does not do its jobs, it could make you unhappy.
Has your poop ever hurt when it's coming out?	(*If yes*) Well, now you know why. It's because your poop was too dry. (*If no*) Good, because that means your poop factory (large intestine)

	is doing its job. It's keeping your poop moist and soft just like you want it to be. The end of your poop factory (large intestine) is called the poop collector (rectum). This is where your poop waits until your body tells you to push it out your poop chute.
Explaining elimination	
You know how a balloon gets bigger when you put air in it?	Well, as your poop collector (rectum) fills up with poop, it starts sending you signals to go to the bathroom. And guess what? The poop collector (rectum) helps the poop factory (large intestine) do one of its two jobs. It also takes water out of your poop.
Does your poop collector (rectum) tell you when you need to poop?	(*If yes*) And what happens if you wait too long to go to the bathroom? That's right. The signal gets stronger and stronger until you have to run to the bathroom. It's just like what happens when you wait too long to pee! (*If no*) That's because poop has stayed in the poop collector too long and it's not able to send you a signal.
What do you think will happen if you cross your legs or squeeze your bottom really hard and don't let your poop come out when it wants to?	That's right; it will stay in your poop collector (rectum).
And what did I say happens to poop if it stays too long in your poop collector (rectum) or in your poop factory (large intestine)?	That's right. It takes more water out of your poop, causing it to become even drier.

Does this make your poop softer or harder?	Harder, that's right.
And is it easy for hard poop to get out your poop chute?	No, you're right!
So, should you hold your poop in or go to the bathroom when you get the signal?	That's right! You should go to the bathroom! What a smart girl you are.

2. "My tummy hurts"

Julie, does your tummy hurt sometimes?	If poop stays in the poop collector (rectum) too long, your belly might stick out and your poop collector (rectum) might send you a signal to go to the bathroom. The signal feels like a tummy ache but it's not coming from your masher (stomach).
	Remember that your masher (stomach) is up here not down here around our/your belly button. So if you get an ache that's around your belly button it might be your poop collector (rectum) telling you that it's full of poop that needs to come out!

3. Poop accidents

Julie, do you sometimes have poop accidents? Do you know why?	It's because poop sometimes sneaks out when you're not thinking about it. Like when you're running, or jumping, or bending over, or when you're holding your breath, or laughing, or when you pass gas!

Do you have poop accidents because you try to hold your poop *in* or because you try to push your poop *out*?	Because you try to hold your poop *in*, that's right!

4. Poop medicines

Do you know why you take a poop medicine (laxative)?	That's right, to help the poop come out.
Do you know how the poop medicine helps your poop come out?	Some poop medicines help your poop come out by not letting your poop factory (large intestine) and your poop collector (rectum) take out too much water. This is the poop medicine that is sometimes mixed in water or juice. It goes into your poop factory (large intestine) and acts like thousands of little sponges that fill up with water and help your poop stay wet and soft. Other poop medicines help your poop come out by making it move faster so that it doesn't have time to become dry and hurt when it comes out. This is the poop medicine that sometimes tastes like root beer or chocolate.
Julie, now you know how your body makes poop!	Don't worry if you forget something. We'll talk about poop again some other time.

10 Poop Medicines That Go In Your Mouth

Oral laxatives

Laxatives are medicines that soften poop and stimulate peristalsis, thereby helping to relieve constipation.

Why are laxatives necessary?

1. To relieve constipation by removing dry hardened poop
2. To keep poop soft and moving through the large intestine
3. To reduce straining when pushing
4. To achieve the goal of having one or two soft but not watery poops each day
5. Because increasing fiber and liquid is not a treatment for functional constipation

Why is continuous laxative use necessary?

1. To allow time for the poop muscle to unlearn the habit of withholding
2. To allow time for the rectum to shrink back to its normal size
3. To allow time for the rectum to regain its normal tone and sensitivity

Water retention laxatives

These are medicines that draw water into the large intestine from the surrounding tissue. This process results in a softer, larger and heavier mass of stool, which stimulates normal bowel action. Table 10.1 has useful information about retention laxatives frequently recommended for childhood constipation.

Table 10.1 Water Retention Laxatives

Laxative Product	Form*	Flavor	Active Ingredient	g/mg
Powderlax® MiraLAX® Laxaclear® Glycolax® and many other brands	powder	tasteless	polyethylene glycol 3350	17g/cap
Pedia-Lax® Chewable	tablet	watermelon	magnesium hydroxide	400mg/tab
Milk of magnesia chewable	tablet	mint	magnesium hydroxide	311mg/tab
Milk of magnesia liquid	liquid	cherry or mint	magnesium hydroxide	400mg/tsp

*Powders should always be mixed in 6-8 oz of fluid. Children who take the tablet or liquid forms of these laxatives should also drink 6-8 oz of fluid.

Polyethylene glycol 3350 (PEG)

PEG is the most commonly recommended water retention laxative for children. Although advertised as tasteless, a surprising number of children say that they do not like the "taste" of PEG powders, even when they are mixed in juice or some other flavored beverage. Here are some tips if your child complains about the taste of "tasteless" powdered laxatives.

How to get children to drink laxatives

1. Mix with cold, sweet, or tart beverages. The colder the better! Cold beverages mask the "taste" of powdered laxatives more effectively than beverages served at room temperature.
2. Your child does not have to drink the laxative all at one time. You may allow up to three to four hours.
3. Mix the powder in less than 8 ounces of liquid. Children sometimes resist taking dissolved laxatives because they do not want "that much" to drink. However, be sure that your child drinks an additional 6 to 8 ounces of liquid within three to four hours after taking the laxative.
4. Mix the powder predissolved in cold foods. Dissolve the required amount of laxative in a few ounces of water before mixing it in a cold food such as ice cream, yogurt or a smoothie. If the powder is not fully dissolved, your child may report a gritty feeling on his tongue and refuse to swallow it.
5. Do not tell your child that you put a laxative in his drink. Deception is the least desirable way to get your child to drink his "poop medicine," but it may be necessary in order to get treatment started.

Negative side effects?

Some but not all children who take water retention laxatives experience stool incontinence, anal irritation, or abdominal cramping. These unwanted effects are sometimes the result of giving more of a laxative than necessary during Steps 2 and 3 of treatment when you and your health care provider are trying to determine the minimum dose necessary to maintain a very soft but not watery stool.

Stimulant laxatives

Stimulant laxatives encourage bowel movements by irritating the inner lining of the intestinal wall. This process increases muscle contractions which move stool toward the rectum. In Table 10.2

you will find useful information about some of the stimulant laxatives that are commonly recommended for children.

Table 10.2 Stimulant Laxatives

Laxative Product	Form*	Flavor	Active Ingredient	g/mg
Ex-lax®	"candy bar"	chocolate	sennosides	15mg/piece
Ex-lax® Regular	pill		sennosides	15mg/pill
Ex-lax® Maximum	pill		sennosides	25mg/pill
Senokot®	tablet		sennosides	8.6mg/tab
Senokot-XTRA®	tablet		sennosides	17.2mg/tab
Fletcher's Laxative® for Kids	liquid	root beer	sennosides	8.8mg/tsp
Dulcolax®	tablet		Bisacodyl	5mg/tab
*All stimulant laxatives should be taken with 6-8 oz of fluid.				

Negative side effects?

Some children who take stimulant laxatives experience stool incontinence, abdominal discomfort or cramps. If a child experiences any of these unwanted side effects it is usually during the Steps 2 and 3 of treatment when you and your doctor are trying to find the laxative and the dose that work best for your child. For this reason, when first introducing any laxative but especially stimulant laxatives, it is best to start with a low dose and then increase the dose gradually until you achieve the desired result.

Are stimulant laxatives safe?

A common misconception about stimulant laxatives is that chemically-stimulated peristalsis will begin to replace natural peristalsis because of damage to intestinal tissue caused by the long-term use of senna-derived laxatives. However, studies over the past 25 years or more have concluded that the long-term use of stimulant laxatives does not cause intestinal damage.[1] Moreover, published findings of clinical research involving large groups of children treated with stimulant laxatives for a year or longer report no peristalsis dependency.[2] Nevertheless, certain usage guidelines are recommended.

Usage guidelines for stimulant laxatives

1. Use the lowest dose possible.
2. Use intermittently if possible.
3. Discontinue if recipient experiences repeated cramping.
4. Limit continuous use to twelve months.

WARNING: Do not exceed the age or length-of-use restrictions in the product directions that come with water retention or stimulant laxatives without the prior approval of your healthcare provider.

Lubricant laxatives

Mineral oil is the most commonly used lubricant laxative. It facilitates bowel movements by coating the large intestine and the stool with a waterproof film which keeps the stool soft and able to move more easily. A lubricant laxative is typically used in large quantities early in the treatment of functional constipation to soften and remove dry, hard stool that is impacted in the rectum.

Negative side effects?

Seepage of mineral oil sometimes occurs when mineral oil is used for cleanouts because of the higher than usual doses often required for cleanouts. Contrary to common thought, long-term use of mineral oil does not cause a vitamin deficiency.[3]

Chapter Notes

1. Wald, A. (2003). Is chronic use of stimulant laxatives harmful to the colon? *Journal of Clinical Gastroenterology*, 36(5), 386–388.
2. Clayden, G. S. (1992). Management of functional constipation. [Personal Practice]. *Archives of Disease in Childhood*, 67, 340–344.
3. Levy, J. and Volpert, D. (2005). Know thy laxatives: A parent's guide to the successful management of chronic functional constipation in infants and children. IFFGD Fact Sheet No. 828, 1–4.

Poop Medicines That Go In Your Poop Chute

11

Enemas and suppositories

Rectal laxatives have been used to relieve constipation since the early 1900s. Even though people today prefer oral laxatives, rectally administered laxatives continue to be used safely and effectively for constipation in children and adults worldwide.

When to consider using a rectal laxative

- If your child's rectum is full of dry, hard stool
- If oral cleanouts have been incomplete or unsuccessful

Unlike in past generations, many adults have never experienced a rectal laxative and just the thought of one makes them feel uneasy. People erroneously think that rectal laxatives hurt, so they are reluctant to use them. If you are extremely anxious about the use of rectal laxatives, do not give one to your child. He will sense your anxiety and be even more anxious and less cooperative than he might have been otherwise.

What if my child resists?

Most children resist rectal laxatives because they think they will hurt. This is especially true for children who, by their temperament, tend to be more anxious or fearful than their peers. If you do decide to give your child a rectal laxative, be extremely patient and allow whatever amount of time, encouragement, and preparation is needed.

Should I force my child?

A child who says "no" to a lot of things may resist a rectal laxative out of stubbornness, fear, or both. Use force only if it is clear that your child's resistance is primarily due to stubbornness. Using force means having one parent gently hold the child while the other parent inserts the laxative. However, if your child puts up strong, physical resistance, you should stop! In the long run, the struggle required is not worth it. Why engage in repeated physical battles at the risk of doing psychological harm when you can accomplish the task with oral laxatives, albeit more slowly and with more leakage.

An Enema Story

It was at the end of a very long road when my wife and I finally made the decision to use enemas to treat our son's encopresis. Looking back, I wish we had done it sooner. The idea was initially suggested by Dr. DuHamel, our child's clinical psychologist. I don't know if it's just our son's personality or if others have had similar results but it turned out to be the most effective of all the treatments we had tried.

Jonas has a very clinical mind. He likes to understand why things happen. This made it easy to explain what we were going to do and why. I told him that holding his poop inside caused his rectum to become stretched, and I used a balloon metaphor to describe what that meant. I told him that if he emptied his balloon every day, it would eventually shrink back to its normal size and he would not have any more accidents. He liked that idea.

My own medical history included many enemas so it was easy for me to explain to him what was going to happen step by step. I believe that Jonas was comforted by knowing that daddy understood how he felt. The first enema was an easy sell. He was much more resistant the second time.

The administration of the enema is only half the battle. It is uncomfortable, but it is over very quickly. I told Jacob that it would be easier for him if he lay on his side with his knees pulled up toward his chest. I explained that I would touch his bottom with the tip of the enema and then, after we counted to three and he exhaled to relax, I would push in the tip of the enema and squeeze in medicine. I took extreme care to never rush him or surprise him. I rubbed his back and just kept telling him how proud I was of him and how excited I was that the enema was going to give him control of his bowels and "fix the balloon."

The penetration was uncomfortable for Jonas but it was when the medicine entered his rectum that he was the most uncomfortable. He squirmed a lot, but luckily he was able to keep the medicine in. I got about two-thirds of the bottle in the first time but, from then on, Jonas wanted to negotiate how much medicine I would put in before he would agree to continue. Even though I told him that the medicine worked better if he stayed on the floor until it began to work, he would immediately sit on the toilet because he was afraid that the poop was going to come out quickly. I was right there with him. I knelt on the floor facing him. He would lean forward a little, lay his head on my shoulder and I would hug him and rub his back the whole time until the big moment.

Jonas was understandably nervous up to this point but it was the outright terror when the medicine started to work that was so surprising to me. He began to cry while screaming, "I can't do this," over and over as the pressure began to build and he began to lose control of his bowels. We had learned from our psychologist that withholding was a "conditioned response" but it was not until this moment that I understood how powerful the conditioning was and how scary the loss of control was for Jonas. I had honestly never seen my child so afraid of anything. Fortunately, it was over quickly.

The look of terror in Jonas' eye was instantly replaced with relief and excitement about what he had just accomplished. It was undoubtedly the first time in a long time that his rectum had been emptied to that extent. Up until this time, even with oral laxatives, he had only let out enough poop to take the pressure off but not enough to empty his rectum. It's hard to remember how long the first enema took from start to finish. I think it was less than one hour but it felt much longer.

With the help of "Dr. Tom," we set up a reward system for pooping on the toilet and told him that it did not matter whether he pooped with the help of the enema or not, he still earned his prize. He was excited about the prize but the prize by itself was not enough to get him to agree to do the second enema. He very matter-of-factly told me, "WE ARE NOT DOING THAT AGAIN!" I said nothing to that and focused on what he had already accomplished so as to keep the moment positive.

The next day we began to negotiate the schedule for future enemas. I wanted Jonas to feel that he was part of the enema decision-making team.

We agreed that now that his balloon was empty, we could not let it overfill again. I knew that Jonas should empty his rectum every day but since he had never had daily bowel movements before (it was not uncommon for him to go many days in a row without having a bowel movement), he and I agreed that we would do an enema every other day—with a couple of stipulations. If he pooped on the potty before his enema, he could skip another day—unless he had an accident in which case he had to have an enema.

It took considerably longer for Jonas to build up his courage the second time. He tried to poop on the toilet a number of times right before his enema. My sense was that this enema was more important than the first because Jonas is strong willed. I knew that if I pushed too hard, we would stalemate. I decided that I was going to stay in the bathroom with him until he was ready. I told him that no matter how long it took, we were both going to stay in the bathroom until he had the enema and pooped in the toilet. After a few false starts and lots of encouragement, Jake finally agreed but he still wanted to negotiate how much of the medicine he would get.

Again, Jonas sat right up on the toilet and we assumed our hugging position. And again there was crying as the medicine began to work but with a little less fear this time—and progressively less each time thereafter. The second enema took over two hours and was by far the longest of them all. As the fear receded, so did the time it took to complete the enema. Toward the end we were able to complete the enema and have a bowel movement within about thirty minutes.

I cannot recall exactly how many enemas we did before Jonas pooped on the toilet naturally but the whole process only took about two weeks. He was SO proud and we were too. He never had a single accident again. • ***Dave K.***

Benefits of rectal laxatives

- Fast, predictable response times
- More certainty about the extent of cleanouts
- Avoids dosing uncertainties of oral laxatives
- Avoids leaking caused by oral laxatives

Preparing your child

A few days prior to your child's first enema or suppository, tell him that you are going to help him get a lot of his poop out by putting poop medicine in his "poop chute." Review the GI tract educational material for children in chapter 9, pointing out where the poop medicine will go and how it makes the poop come out.

Next, if you use an enema, show your child the container used to put the medicine into his poop chute. Emphasize how little water there is in the container and how the tip of the container is so small and slippery. Encourage him to hold the container and push out the water as if was a squirt gun. Show him how to refill the container with tap water and give him permission to play with it as much as he wants. Likewise, if you use a solid suppository, let him feel how slippery it is and how quickly it melts in his hand.

Now take him to the room where the enema/suppository will be administered (usually the bathroom). Get down on the floor yourself to demonstrate the two most common positions (Figure 11.1), and then ask him to lie on the floor and get into the position he prefers. Two or more additional "rehearsals" with pants off, so that his buttocks are bare, should help him relax during the actual procedure.

The positions most often recommended when giving an enema to children are to lie on their left side with one or both knees bent up toward their chest or to lie on their stomach with both knees pulled up to their chest.

Figure 11.1 Enema Positions

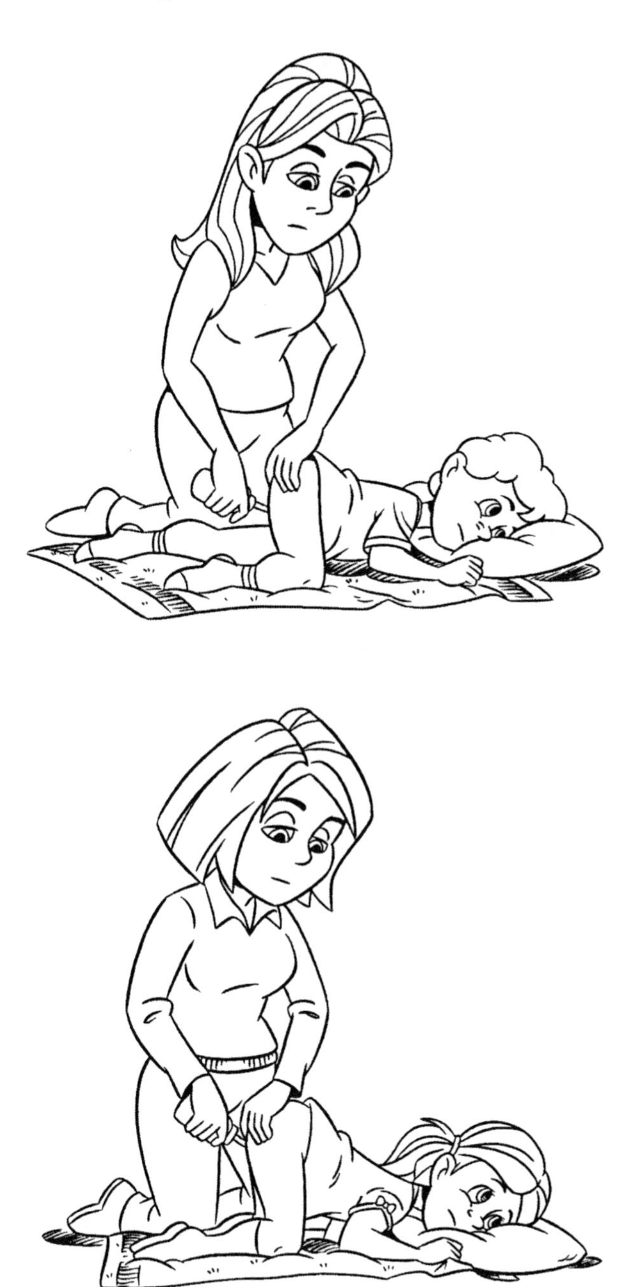

Which enema or suppository should I use?

Enemas

An enema is a procedure for introducing water and other stimulating substances into the lower intestinal tract via the anus. The increasing volume of liquid causes a rapid expansion of the rectum resulting in a strong and fairly rapid urge to poop. Enemas containing sodium phosphate (saline) are preferable because they cause little or no anal irritation. Products used with children include:

- Pedia-Lax® (saline) enema
- Fleet® (saline) enema

Liquid suppositories

Like an enema, a liquid suppository is a procedure for putting medicine into the rectum where it stimulates nerve endings causing muscle contractions and a strong, rapid urge to poop. Glycerin suppositories are recommended for children because they are gentle on the GI tract. Products for children include:

- Pedia-Lax® Liquid Glycerin Suppository
- Fleet® Liquid Glycerin Suppository

Solid suppositories

A solid suppository is a drug-delivery system consisting of a small missile-shaped medicine preparation that is inserted into the rectum via the anus where it melts and releases the medicine. Products for children include:

- Pedia-Lax® Glycerin Suppository
- Fleet® Glycerin Suppository

How to give your child a rectal laxative

Ask your child to lie on a large towel placed on the bathroom floor, and have him assume his preferred position. Go slowly and talk reassuringly. Do not rush. Place a pillow under his head to help him feel more comfortable. It is sometimes easier for a child to relax in this situation if he is allowed to watch his favorite DVD, play a hand-held video game, or engage in some other favorite activity.

If he is lying on his stomach with both knees pulled up, hold the enema bottle with one hand and separate his buttocks with your other hand until you can see the anal opening. If he is lying on his side, place your other hand gently on his upper buttock and lift it so that you can find the anal opening.

When giving an enema be sure that the liquid is at or slightly above room temperature. It is sometimes easier for a child to hold in the liquid if the container has been warmed beforehand, just as you would warm a baby's bottle. Before inserting the tip of the enema or liquid suppository, ask your child to slowly breathe in and out a few times and then ask him to "push" as if he were trying to have a bowel movement. Deep breathing and pushing sometimes help relax the anal sphincter making insertion easier. Simultaneously with your child's deep breathing and/or pushing, slowly insert the lubricated tip of the enema/liquid suppository into your child's anal opening in the direction of his belly button using a slight side-to-side motion.

When giving a solid suppository, use one finger to push either the narrow end or the blunt end into your child's anus. Sometimes, when the blunt or back end of the suppository goes in first, it seems to get sucked in more easily. Solid suppositories melt quickly so do not pick one up until you are ready to insert it. Push the suppository in the direction of your child's belly button far enough to get past the anal sphincter, typically 1 to 1½ inches for children. Use your index finger and push the suppository up to or a little past the first knuckle. If the suppository slips back out, you did not push it in far enough. You may have to try again with a new suppository if the first one is too slippery.

Caution: If your child squeezes his buttocks together so tightly that excessive force is necessary to insert the tip of the enema/liquid suppository or the solid suppository, stop and reassure him that it will not hurt before trying again.

Enemas and suppositories usually take five to ten minutes to be maximally effective. Ask your child to stay in a horizontal position and, if necessary, squeeze his buttocks together to help prevent the laxative and/or stool from coming out too soon. When held in long enough, rectal laxatives will empty only one-quarter of a 5-foot-long colon which is why a second enema within hours of the first enema may be necessary for an effective cleanout.

Knees Up, Belly Button In

12

Sitting and pushing

Sitting and pushing correctly increases the likelihood of a successful bowel movement. This is true for everyone but especially for children who are constipated. If your child needs some extra encouragement to sit and push when asked, use an incentive system like the one described in Example 1 in Chapter 13.

How to sit

1. Have buttocks and tailbone well supported, not hanging down
2. Have feet flat on the floor or stool with knees slightly above buttocks
3. Lean slightly forward from the waist
4. Spread insides of knees 5 to 10 inches apart, depending on age

Toddlers who have outgrown their potty chair will need a toilet seat insert in order to sit on the toilet correctly. An insert that fits snugly and has handles works best, just in case your child has a fear of falling off or into the toilet. Handles also help a child push properly by providing leverage.

When to sit

Encourage your child to sit whenever he says or acts like he needs to pee or poop. The best time for a child to sit and "try" to poop (even if he says he doesn't have to) is within 10 to 15 minutes of

Figure 12.1 Sitting Posture

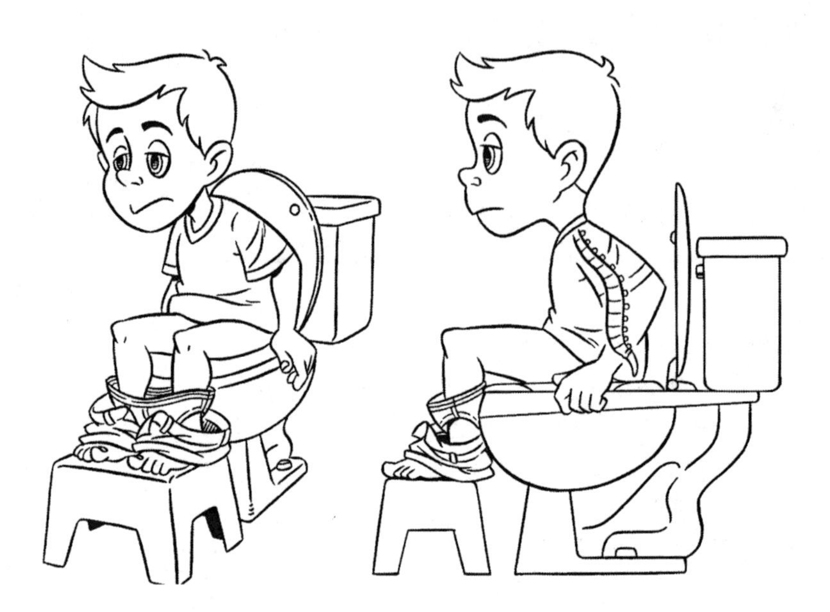

eating in order to take advantage of the gastrocolic reflex. Recall that this reflex is strongest in the morning, so sitting after breakfast is encouraged provided that your child is not rushed. Stress makes it more difficult to pee or poop. Have your child sit and "try to poop" after two or three meals each day. He does not need to sit at school (of course he can if he wants to) but he should sit following after-school snack. In fact, this is often one of the most successful "sits" of the day.

If your child has a bowel movement early in the day, ask him to sit again later in the day, particularly if he has had something to eat in the interim. It is amazing how much poop children are able to produce in one day!

How long to sit?

When a child is asked to sit to try to poop after a meal or snack, he should sit until he has completed the sitting sequence (explained later in this chapter) three times. Of course, if he produces a medium to large poop at any time during his sit, even if it occurs within the first few minutes; do not require that he sit any longer. But if it is only a small poop, he should sit until he passes more poop (children often have two bowel movements in one sitting) or until he has pushed six times. This is the ideal scenario. The reality of "sits" is often quite different.

When to stop sitting

Sitting to try to poop is not the way most children choose to spend their time, particularly children with functional constipation. Incentives are frequently necessary to motivate a child to sit for this length of time. However, even with incentives there will be times when your child digs in his heels and says, "No!" When this happens, do not get into a battle over sitting. Simply say, "Okay, we'll do it later." Even if you are able to drag him into the bathroom and get him to sit on the toilet, it is unlikely that he will be able to relax enough to pass stool.

Parent participation

I strongly recommend that parents be in the bathroom when their child is trying to poop. Parental participation is critical for keeping a child focused and motivated by doing things with him that he enjoys. Your job is to help your child relax and to encourage him to push as instructed. If you are impatient or resentful of having to spend your time helping him do something that you think he is old enough to do by himself, it will just be that much more difficult for him to relax.

What should I expect?

It is unrealistic to think that your child is going to have a bowel movement every time he sits on the toilet to poop. Think of each sit as an opportunity for your child to practice pushing and to feel relaxed while sitting on the toilet. If he passes stool, congratulate him. If he does not, praise him for trying. Always keep in mind that the treatment of functional constipation is a marathon, not a sprint. If you get discouraged, so will your child.

Pushing

When severely constipated children sit on the toilet to try to poop, some of them push correctly, but others only act like they are pushing. Some children just sit there and wait for the poop to come out. This is also true for children who poop in their diapers or Pull-ups outside of the bathroom. In some cases, sitting and waiting for poop to come out is related to withholding. However, many children simply do not know how to push. They must be taught.

Pushing Instructions

1. "Inhale a little and hold it."
2. "Pull in your belly button a little and hold it in."
3. "Try to push your belly button down and out through your poop chute." *(The muscle below the belly button should be hard.)*
4. "Push for three to five seconds; then exhale and relax."

Pushing Pointers

- Begin by having your child sit on the toilet and asking him to pee.
- Relaxing the urinary sphincter helps relax the anal sphincter.
- If he is able to pee, ask him to start pushing while he is peeing.
- Do not pressure him if he is unable to pee or is unwilling to try.

Pushing sequence

Ask your child to push for five seconds, think for fifteen seconds, push again for five seconds, and then rest.

- Do not let your child push too hard. A red face is unnecessary.
- "Think" means to "listen quietly for your body's signals that poop is coming."
- "Rest" means a brief (two to three minutes) fun time with parent, e.g., reading, talking.

Repeat the sequence

Have your child repeat the sequence three times (6 pushes) before ending the sit.

- You may vary the length of the rest periods to maintain attention and focus.
- Stop the sit if your child begins to resist.

Delayed response

Do not be surprised if your child passes stool within five to ten minutes after sitting—a common occurrence, especially early in treatment. This happens when your child's poop muscle doesn't relax until he gets off the toilet and moves away from the bathroom. With time he will be able to relax while sitting on the toilet, and these after-sit accidents will stop. Until then, you might occasionally try having him return to the bathroom within three to five minutes to "try again."

13 Honey Makes the Medicine Go Down

Incentives

Emilie was 9 years old and had been struggling with functional constipation for more than five years when her parents first brought her in to see me. In an initial meeting with Emilie and her parents, Emilie said that she was tired of having accidents and that she wished that they would just go away. At the end of our meeting, I asked Emilie if she would be willing to sit on the toilet every day after breakfast and dinner and try to poop. She said that she would.

The following conversation took place in my office two weeks later.

> **Father to me:** *Emilie has been very good about taking her laxative this past week but not about sitting on the toilet after meals. She says that she doesn't want to sit, so we have to tell her to sit. If she really does want to stop having accidents, why doesn't she sit on her own? Why do her mother and I always have to tell her to do it?*
>
> **Father to Emilie:** *Emilie, why won't you sit on the toilet unless your mother and I tell you to do it?*
>
> **Emilie:** *I don't know; I just don't want to.*

> **I said to Emilie:** *Emilie, can you think of any reason why you don't want to sit on the toilet after you eat?*
>
> **Emilie:** *Well, yeah, it takes too long and it's boring.*

Emilie's dad was understandably confused and frustrated by his daughter's answer. Parents of school-aged children just assume that their child will take responsibility for managing their poop problem and are understandably disappointed when they do not.

Why incentives are necessary

The treatment of functional constipation requires almost nonstop parental encouragement. Some of the reasons for this have to do with a child's age, level of maturity, and temperament. Incentives are needed because so many of the things we ask these children to do day after day are repetitive and boring. A child is no more likely to voluntarily sit on the toilet after every meal than he is to voluntarily do his chores.

How to use incentives effectively

Young children

Money motivates adults, but it rarely motivates preschoolers. Stars, stickers, and small prizes are more effective. To find an effective incentive for your preschooler, think about things she likes to do, such as playing with Legos or small action figures. You might make playing with these toys, or earning new ones, contingent on doing what you want her to do. Small inexpensive prizes are better for ongoing treatment than big, expensive ones. Most parents are able to come up with incentives that do not require daily trips to the toy store. I have found this to be true even for parents who tell me that there is *nothing* that will motivate their child.

Siblings and Incentives

Our son, Tyler, is a 4 ½-year-old boy with a "pleaser" personality sprinkled with drama and stubbornness. Early in his treatment for constipation, we learned that the reason he did not go to the potty on his own and required frequent reminders was because he could not "feel" when he had to go. However, after months of treatment including a significant decrease in laxatives, we began to suspect that he did have the physical ability to control his bowels but was choosing not to.

We affirmed our suspicions when we went out of town with him for nine days and he had zero potty accidents. In nearly every instance, Tyler was able to tell us he needed to go and be completely responsible for getting to the potty. After returning from vacation, he immediately reverted back to refusing to stop playing to go to the potty. Hence, we initiated an incentive system of earning stickers for each time he successfully alerted us to his need to poop and made it to the potty on time. He had to earn four stickers to get a meaningful reward such as watching a new or favorite movie. He lost a sticker every time he had a potty accident.

As usual Tyler's twin brother wanted in on the system, and it quickly became a competition of who had the most stickers. We needed to add other behaviors to the system, such as getting dressed, in order to make it a fair competition. Tyler was consumed by the competitive aspect of it and cared less about the actual reward. His brother, on the other hand, wanted the big prize and worried less about beating Tyler. In fact, he encouraged Tyler so they could watch the movie together. Tyler would count his stickers in the morning and, as a result, our reminders changed from "Do you need to go potty?" to "How many stickers do you need to do [XYZ]?" • ***Krista P.***

Home-Baked Cookies

Simon, our rather bright and stubborn four year old, was resisting his transition to pooping in the toilet. We had been giving him candy sprinkles as an incentive, though the novelty of that approach was quickly wearing off. While I was nursing Simon's younger brother at bedtime, I could hear Simon making various pre-pooping noises. I reminded him of the tasty sprinkles that were awaiting him if he pooped in the toilet. He informed me he would just poop in his diaper tonight.

Afraid that the progress we had made in the last week or two would be lost, I remembered that we still had a home-baked cookie in our kitchen. I reminded Simon of that cookie. "If you poop in the toilet instead of your diaper," I told him, "you could have half of that cookie." That sounded like a good idea to him. He deposited his modest poop in the toilet and received his half cookie (after washing his hands, of course). Then he went to bed.

A short time after this, he told me that he felt another poop coming. I dangled the remaining half-cookie as an incentive. It worked! He pooped again in the toilet. As he was finishing up the second half-cookie reward, he felt a third poop coming on. "I'll just poop in my diaper this time, Mommy. "We're all out of cookies." And so he did. • ***Leigh T.***

Older children

Finding incentives that work with older children can be a challenge. Some are motivated by being able to accumulate screen time for each star they earn during the day, an effective incentive provided it is the only way they can get screen time. Others are motivated by being able to turn in their stars for small amounts of money which they can either spend right away or save for a future purchase. Of course, offering money in return for cooperation only works if a child has no other source of money such as an allowance or their "savings."

Charts and checklists

Parents and teachers will frequently use star charts or check lists to reward compliance. Implemented correctly, charts and lists can be effective motivational tools. They are ineffective if implemented incorrectly. This is why some parents who have not had success with charts or lists erroneously conclude that they do not work.

In order to set up an effective incentive system for changing an established behavior or for teaching a new behavior, you need to know a few of the basic rules of positive reinforcement.

Rules of positive reinforcement

1. *Immediate* positive reinforcement leads to faster learning than delayed positive reinforcement.
2. *Frequent* positive reinforcement leads to faster learning than infrequent positive reinforcement.
3. *Labeled* positive reinforcement leads to faster learning than unlabeled positive reinforcement.

Labeled means that children are told specifically what they did to earn a star. For example, if a child *willingly* took her laxative, you would say, "Thank you for taking your poop medicine right when I asked you to." This is preferable to simply saying, "Thank you." It is important to reinforce *both* of the things your child did that pleased you. She not only took her laxative, she took it quickly and without resistance.

Say "thank you" like you mean it!

All children want to please their parents even though it might not always look that way. When a child knows that her parents are happy about something she has done for them, it makes her feel good. In other words, parental pleasure is positively reinforcing. When expressed convincingly, parental pleasure can be a very powerful and long-lasting incentive. By convincingly, I mean with a big smile, some enthusiasm and an occasional "high five" or a hug for being especially cooperative.

Why children lose interest

One reason children lose interest in stars or stickers is because their parents mistakenly believe that it is the star or sticker that reinforces and sustains their child's motivation. However, the best reinforcement is actually the stickers *combined* with the positive interaction that takes place each time a sticker is earned and placed on the chart. Therefore, to maximize the effectiveness of stars, stickers and prizes, always have your child with you when you place a star or sticker on her chart so that she can see, hear, and *feel* how pleased you are about what she did for you.

Children also lose interest because they get bored with the same rewards day after day, even if their parents are enthusiastic about giving them. That is why it is a good idea to offer different kinds of stickers or prizes from time to time to maintain your child's interest. When you shop for stickers and other small prizes, you can save yourself a lot of guess work and increase the likelihood that your child will work for what you buy, if you take her along with you so she can show you exactly which ones she likes.

Guidelines for setting up charts and checklists

1. ***The list of desired tasks should be short.***
   You can add to it later. Parents have a tendency to create a "laundry list" of tasks which can overwhelm a child and cause them to lose interest quickly. Your child is more likely to finish a short list than a long one.

2. ***The list should include more easy tasks than hard tasks.***
   Hard tasks are tasks that your child has never done before or has never done voluntarily. You want your child to look at the list and think to herself that it is going to be easy to get the stars or checks. If she thinks this way, she will be more likely to do a hard task along with the easy ones in order to get a

bigger reward.

3. ***Clearly define behavioral goals for your child.***
   Do not assume that she knows exactly what it is that you want her to do. For example, instead of saying, "Please do your chores," you should say, "Please empty the trash and feed the dog."

4. ***Follow the rule of "successive approximations."***
   If there is a goal that you want your child to achieve that involves multiple steps (the equivalent of going from A to Z), reinforce some of the intermediate steps in order to increase the likelihood that she will reach Z. For example, if you want your daughter to use good table manners, such as not interrupting when someone else is talking or using her fork or spoon rather than her fingers, praise her multiple times for doing each of these things throughout the meal rather than waiting until the end of the meal to praise her once for using good manners.

Example 1: Pushing

Severely constipated children often need to be taught to "push" in order to have a bowel movement. Some don't push properly. Others have to re-learn because they stopped pushing in order to avoid pain. Demonstrating how to push and then having a child practice it once or twice is not enough to be certain that she has learned how to do it or that she will do it every time she sits to try to poop. Instructions for pushing are in Chart 1. Note that the instructions begin by having a child urinate. Relaxing the muscle that controls urination makes it easier to relax the muscle that controls pooping.

Chart 1. Good Pushing Chart

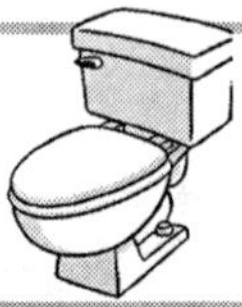

AMELIA'S GOOD PUSHING CHART

INSTRUCTION	SUN	MON	TUE	WED	THU	FRI	SAT
1. TRY TO PEE	☺	☺	☺	☺	☺	☺	☺
2. BREATHE IN SLIGHTLY AND HOLD IT	☺	☺	☺	☺	☺	☺	☺
3. PULL IN YOUR BELLY BUTTON		☺	☺	☺	☺	☺	☺
4. HARDEN THE MUSCLES BELOW YOUR BELLY BUTTON		☺	☺	☺	☺	☺	☺
5. TRY TO PUSH YOUR BELLY BUTTON OUT YOUR "POOP CHUTE"				☺	☺	☺	☺

Test your knowledge: Teaching a child to push is best accomplished with a daily incentive system that incorporates the chart guidelines and positive reinforcement rules described earlier. See if you can figure out which of these guidelines and rules Amelia's parents used to create their daughter's "Good Pushing" chart.

If you identified any of these elements on Amelia's chart, good for you.

☑ Chart guidelines:

1. The list is short.
2. Three of the four tasks are easy.
3. "Good pushing" has been clearly defined.
4. Successive approximations to pushing are reinforced.

☑ Positive reinforcement rules:

1. Reinforcement is immediate.
2. Reinforcement is given frequently.
3. Each task is "labeled."

Example 2: Daily bowel movements

Chart 2 clearly defines and gives a child immediate and frequent positive reinforcement for doing those tasks which increase the likelihood that she will reach her goal of one or more large bowel movements a day.

This chart was created for a child named Matthew by his parents. When creating a chart for your child, incorporate details specific to your child's treatment plan. For example, a child may not be asked to sit after lunch when in school but instead be asked to sit following his or her after-school snack.

Chart 2. Good Pooping Chart

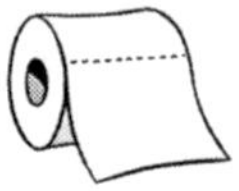

MATTHEW'S GOOD POOPING CHART

INSTRUCTION	SUN	MON	TUE	WED	THU	FRI	SAT
1. TAKE POOP MEDICINE	☆	☆	☆	☆	☆	☆	☆
2. SIT FOR AT LEAST 5 MINUTES AFTER EATING							
▸ BREAKFAST		☆	☆	☆	☆	☆	☆
▸ LUNCH	☆	☆	☆	☆	☆	☆	☆
▸ DINNER	☆	☆	☆	☆	☆	☆	☆
3. PUSH 6 TIMES DURING EACH SITTING							
▸ BREAKFAST			☆	☆	☆	☆	
▸ LUNCH		☆	☆	☆	☆	☆	☆
▸ DINNER		☆	☆	☆	☆	☆	☆
4. PEE IN TOILET (1 STAR EACH TIME)	☆	☆ ☆ ☆	☆ ☆	☆ ☆ ☆ ☆	☆ ☆ ☆	☆ ☆ ☆ ☆	☆ ☆ ☆
5. POOP IN TOILET (3 STARS EACH TIME)				☆ ☆ ☆	☆ ☆ ☆ ☆ ☆ ☆		☆ ☆ ☆ ☆ ☆ ☆

Note: Encourage boys to sit to pee at least twice/day.

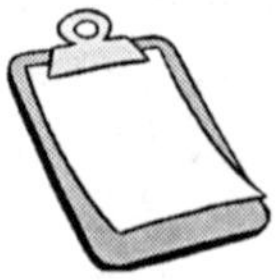

Example 3: Poop while sitting on the toilet

As mentioned earlier, some children are afraid to sit on the toilet to poop. Most of them have poop "accidents" in their underwear. Since these girls and boys are usually not afraid to sit on the toilet to urinate, sitting to pee is a task that is always included on their charts. In addition to being a close approximation to pooping on the toilet, relaxing the pee muscle also helps relax the poop muscle, thereby increasing the likelihood that pushing will be successful.

Chart 3 should be explained to your child as an opportunity to "practice" sitting on the toilet, along with the assurance that it is okay if she doesn't poop. Parents should be forewarned that accidents can happen at this stage. In fact, it is not uncommon for a child to finish practicing and then, shortly thereafter, have a bowel movement in her underwear. This sort of accident can occur because her rectal muscle will begin to relax as soon as she moves away from the toilet.

Chart 3. Good Sitting on the Toilet to Poop Chart

REBECCA'S GOOD SITTING ON THE TOILET CHART

INSTRUCTION	SUN	MON	TUE	WED	THU	FRI	SAT
1. SIT ON TOILET (3–5 MIN) WITH CLOTHES ON	☺☺☺	☺☺☺	☺☺	☺	☺		
2. SIT ON TOILET (3–5 MIN) WITH UNDERWEAR ON		☺	☺☺	☺☺	☺		
3. SIT ON TOILET (3–5 MIN) WITH BARE BOTTOM	☺		☺☺	☺	☺☺	☺☺	☺☺
4. SIT ON TOILET TO PEE*	☺		☺	☺☺	☺☺☺	☺☺☺☺	☺☺☺☺
5. SIT ON TOILET AND PUSH TO TRY TO POOP	☺		☺	☺	☺	☺☺	☺☺

Remember, additional positive reinforcement for a task that is more difficult increases the likelihood that a child will try to do that task.

Example 4: Diapers and Pull-ups

Parents find it difficult to change the behavior of children who have become dependent on, and will only *poop* in, a diaper or a Pull-up. It's even more difficult to change the behavior of children who will only *pee and poop* in a diaper or Pull-up. The treatment of these children occurs in three different phases.

- Phase 1. Teach them to poop/pee in the bathroom while wearing a diaper or Pull-up.
- Phase 2. Teach them to poop/pee sitting on the toilet while wearing a diaper or Pull-up.
- Phase 3. Teach them to poop/pee sitting on the toilet without a diaper or Pull-up.

■ Phase 1

The goal by the end of Phase 1 is to have the child routinely poop/pee in one "spot" in the bathroom. Recall that because these children wear diapers and Pull-ups, they can poop in any room they choose. Many of them go to a "secret" location or spot to poop such as under the dining room table or behind the living room sofa.

At the beginning of this phase, identify and mark the spot or spots where your child routinely poops or pees by putting masking tape or some other material on the floor at the spot. Create an "X" or some other shape such as a smiley face on the spot. Then add several new "spots" in the direction of the bathroom. Place one spot close to where the child already poops or pees and two or three others in locations that are progressively closer to the bathroom. Put the last spot just inside the bathroom door. By placing the spot progressively closer to the bathroom, you are following the rule of successive approximations—one of the four guidelines for setting up charts and checklists.

Chart 4. Good Pooping on the Spot Chart

LUCA'S GOOD POOPING ON THE SPOT CHART

INSTRUCTION	SUN	MON	TUE	WED	THU	FRI	SAT
1. STAND ON A SPOT AFTER YOU POOP OR PEE (1 STAR EACH TIME)	★	★	★★	★★★	★★★★	★★★★	★★★★
2. STAND ON A SPOT WHILE YOU POOP OR PEE (1 STAR EACH TIME)				★★	★★★	★★★★	★★★★
3. STAND ON A SPOT CLOSER TO THE BATHROOM TO POOP (2 STARS EACH TIME)						★★	★★
4. STAND ON THE SPOT INSIDE THE BATHROOM TO POOP (3 STARS EACH TIME)					★★★		★★★★★★

In this example, because a child urinates and sometimes poops more than once a day, the amount of positive reinforcement he can earn adds up quickly. This takes advantage of the fact that immediate and frequent positive reinforcements are more motivating and, therefore, lead to faster learning.

■ Phase 2

Once a child is able to poop and pee routinely in a diaper or Pull-up while standing in the bathroom, she is ready to move to an incentive chart that is a variation of Chart 3. This chart will help to motivate her to sit on the toilet while wearing her diaper or Pull-up and may even be sufficient to motivate her to go directly from wearing a diaper or Pull-up to not wearing anything while sitting on the toilet.

Chart 5. Good Sitting on the Toilet Chart

☺ JACKIE'S GOOD SITTING ON THE TOILET CHART							
INSTRUCTION	SUN	MON	TUE	WED	THU	FRI	SAT
1. SIT ON TOILET (3-5 MIN) WITH DIAPERS OR PULL-UPS ON		✔	✔✔	✔✔	✔	✔✔✔✔	✔✔✔✔
2. SIT ON TOILET (3-5 MIN) WITH BARE BOTTOM	✔		✔✔	✔	✔✔	✔✔	✔✔
3. SIT ON TOILET TO PEE*	✔		✔	✔✔	✔✔✔	✔✔✔✔	✔✔✔✔
4. SIT ON TOILET AND PUSH TO TRY TO POOP	✔		✔	✔	✔	✔✔	✔✔

Note: Encourage boys to sit to pee at least twice/day.

■ Phase 3

Many children find it extremely difficult to poop or pee without a diaper or Pull-up on. Wearing a diaper or Pull-up helps them relax their poop and pee muscles, in part by assuring them that their poop or pee will not drop into the toilet. For these children, diapers and Pull-ups give a sense of security or comfort much like children experience with a "security blanket." Therefore, the incentive chart that these children need is one that focuses specifically on their diaper or Pull-up dependency.

Chart 6. Good Sitting on the Toilet in a Diaper Chart

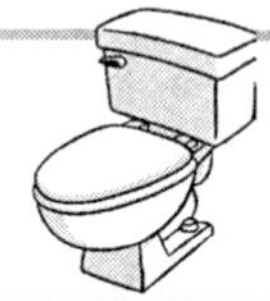

KEATON'S GOOD SITTING ON THE TOILET IN A DIAPER CHART

INSTRUCTION	SUN	MON	TUE	WED	THU	FRI	SAT
1. PRACTICE SITTING ON TOILET WITH DIAPER ON	X X	X	X X	X X			
2. PEE/POOP ON TOILET WITH DIAPER ON			X X	X			
3. PEE/POOP WITH SMALL SLIT IN DIAPER				X X	X X X		X X X X
4. PEE/POOP ON TOILET WITH VERY SMALL HOLE IN DIAPER					X	X X	
5. PEE/POOP ON TOILET WITH LARGER HOLE IN DIAPER							
6. PEE/POOP WITH NO DIAPER							

Note: Substitute "Pull-up" for diaper when appropriate.

This incentive chart includes more steps than other charts because most diaper-dependent children will refuse to pee or poop if they perceive the cut in their diaper to be too big. Therefore, each successive slit or hole in the diaper can only be slightly larger than the one preceding it. Even with this, many children stay with a very small opening (slit) for weeks or months before they feel comfortable enough to progress to a slightly larger opening. In fact, there are some children who continue to "need" their diaper even after it is nothing more than a belt around their waist.

The Diaper Belt

Once again, my daughter climbed off the toilet without having had success even though I knew she had to go. I also knew that if I let her put on a diaper, she would go. Why was she able to go in a diaper but not in the toilet? As an experienced mother of four, I knew that this was not a power struggle. Something else was going on here.

Then, one day after drinking a lot of water and sitting on the toilet longer than usual, she actually peed! I was elated and I thought she would be thrilled. She was not. In fact, her face registered terror rather than triumph. It was at that moment that I first realized that my daughter was afraid to go unless she was wearing a diaper.

Our journey began with a referral to a psychologist who specialized in children with elimination problems. When we first began to work with Dr. Tom, I was very curious to know what he would suggest that I had not already tried. Sticker charts? Been there. Special rewards? Done that. But after working together for a while, he suggested a tactic that proved to be the key to unlocking the door to my daughter's fears. It was a long slow process that tested my patience to its limits but, in the end, it was worth it. My daughter no longer needed to wear a diaper to poop or pee.

We began by having her practice sitting on her potty chair with her diaper on. She did not have to poop or pee. The potty chair didn't even need to be in the bathroom. Initially, she got a sticker for just sitting on the potty but, in time, with a lot of encouragement, she got stickers for peeing or pooping into her diaper while sitting on her potty chair. Eventually, because she was now 5 years old, she outgrew the potty chair. It was time to graduate to the toilet with a potty seat and a stool for her feet. We again gave her stickers just for sitting. It felt like back-

tracking at first, but since nothing else had worked, I persevered. In time she began to earn rewards for pooping or peeing in her diaper while seated on the toilet. She got one sticker for sitting, two more for peeing and, if she pooped, she hit pay dirt: five stickers! And as soon as she reached a set number of stickers, she got a small toy.

Next came the part that really began to challenge her. At Dr. Tom's suggestion, I explained to her that we were going to cut a small slit in the center of her diaper near the back. She became anxious about this and required a lot of reassurance. When it was time to use the toilet she put on a diaper with a slit in it, sat on the toilet, and tried to go. At first, she was reluctant, but she became more comfortable when she realized that it was rare that anything actually made it through the slit into the toilet. She began to lose interest in the stickers so we purchased a toy set that she wanted that had many pieces (Polly Pockets). Now, when successful, she could choose to have a small piece of the set or save up her stickers to earn a larger piece.

After several months we began to make the slit larger and then gradually widened it into a hole. She was told each time we were going to increase the size of the hole. If she showed too much anxiety, we would wait. It was often three or more weeks before we could move up to a larger hole. As time went by, her resistance to enlarging the hole lessened but the need to have the diaper continued.

She was past her sixth birthday when the realization struck her. We had progressed along with our ever growing hole, going from a hole that was big enough for all of her poop and pee to pass through, to a diaper cut so close that only the elastic leg and waist bands were touching her and, finally, to what we called the "diaper belt." Dr. Tom told her that she could wear her diaper belt all the time if she liked, but she preferred to put it on just

> *before sitting on the toilet.*
>
> *At this point I had gone from irritation at my daughter's inability to perform on the toilet to amusement that she somehow had not yet discovered the truth of her situation. It was one day about three weeks after she was regularly using her diaper belt when she looked up at me and declared gravely, 'You know, Mom, I don't think this diaper belt is doing anything." I tried to hide my enormous grin out of respect for her seriousness and responded, "You know, I think you are right."* • ***Erica G.***

Punishment

By the time parents reach the point of seeking professional help for their child's constipation, they have usually tried everything they can think of to correct the problem, including punishment. This is understandable since punishment, or simply the threat of punishment, can be an effective motivator. For example, you might tell your child that she will not get any dessert unless she eats everything on her plate. However, when used to get a child to poop on the toilet, punishment is rarely, if ever, effective. In fact, when used to motivate severely constipated children, punishment is counterproductive and can be psychologically harmful.

Severely constipated children are unable to poop or to stop having accidents on demand. They are at the mercy of their dysfunctional lower GI tract. Punishing a child for not pooping on the toilet and for having accidents is punishing her for something she cannot do and cannot control. The threat of being punished for not pooping on the toilet actually makes it harder for a child to poop because she becomes stressed and is, therefore, less able to relax her poop muscle.

Young children, whether constipated or not, believe that their parents know everything. That is why children ask their parents so many questions. So, when a parent emphatically tells a child to poop on the toilet, the child believes that she should be able to do it. If she is successful, great! However, if she is repeatedly unsuccessful, she begins to think that there must be something wrong with her and that, since she cannot please her parents, she must not be a likable or lovable child. Over time, this thinking can lead to a poor self image and lack of self esteem.

Food and Drink for Good Poops

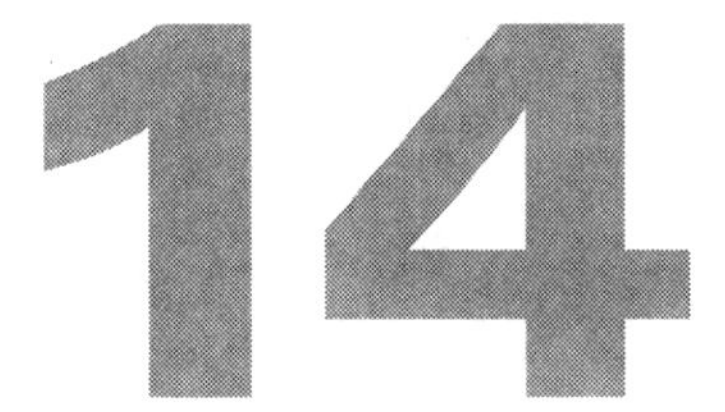

Fiber and liquids

Diets low in fiber or liquid do not cause functional constipation. Functional constipation is caused by stool withholding and subsequent rectal distention. Studies that have attempted to treat functional constipation by increasing dietary fiber and/or liquids have not demonstrated significant benefit.[1] However, for prevention, fiber-rich diets are recommended for all children, especially those who have a history of occasional or functional constipation.

Dietary fiber

Dietary fiber is defined as indigestible carbohydrates found in plant cell walls. There are two types of fiber, soluble and insoluble. Soluble fiber dissolves in water and becomes a soft gel. Insoluble fiber does not dissolve in water. It absorbs water, which adds bulk to the stool. Soluble fiber slows transit time in the small intestine allowing nutrients to be absorbed more efficiently. Insoluble fiber promotes regularity by slowing transit time in the large intestine so it can absorb water and bulk.

Soluble and insoluble fiber

Dietary sources of fiber typically contain both types of fiber, but soluble and insoluble fiber is more concentrated in some foods than in others. (See Table 14.1)

Table 14.1 Foods High in Fiber

Soluble Fiber	Insoluble Fiber
Oats	Wheat bran
Barley	Whole grain breads
Soy beans	Vegetables
Peas	Dried beans
Citrus fruit	Popcorn
	Brown rice

Fiber and liquid daily requirements

Adult consumption of fiber in the United States is estimated to be 15 grams of fiber daily which is far below the recommended daily adult goal of 25 grams for adult women and 38 grams for adult men.[2] For children the amount of fiber recommended is "the age of the child plus 5 grams." For example, a 3-year-old child should consume 9 grams of fiber daily. Dietitians recommend that at least one-fourth of total fiber come from sources rich in soluble fiber.

Recommended liquid consumption from all sources for children 1 to 8 years of age is 4 to 5 cups (32 to 40 fluid ounces). For children 9 to 13 years of age, consumption of 7 to 8 cups (56-64 fluid ounces) from all sources is recommended.[3]

The Nutrition Facts printed on most food packaging tells you how much dietary fiber the product contains per serving. Some nutrition labels also break down the total into soluble and insoluble. If the label shows only soluble fiber, you can determine the amount of insoluble fiber by subtracting that number from the total. Our digestive system needs both types of fiber but insoluble fiber contributes more to stool regularity because of its water absorption or bulking action in the large intestine. Figure 14.2

shows a sample Nutrition Facts label from a box of cereal.

Figure 14.2 Sample Nutrition Facts Label

Nutrition Facts

Serving Size 1 1/4 cup (59g)
Servings per Container about 9

Amount Per Serving	Cereal	Cereal with ½ cup Fat Free Milk
Calories	200	240
Calories from Fat	10	10
	% Daily Value	
Total Fat 1g	2%	2%
Saturated Fat 0g	0%	0%
Trans Fat 0g		
Polyunsaturated Fat 0.5g		
Monounsaturated Fat 0g		
Cholesterol 0mg	0%	0%
Sodium 0mg	0%	3%
Potassium 230mg	7%	12%
Total Carbohydrate 49g	16%	18%
Dietary Fiber 9g	32%	32%
Soluble Fiber 1g		
Insoluble Fiber 7g		
Sugars <1g		
Other Carbohydrate 40g		
Protein 6g		

Fiber supplements

Fiber supplements can be made from natural or synthetic sources. The leading brands use a range of different fibers in their products; the most common of these is psyllium, a soluble fiber plant. As with laxatives, particular supplements tend to work better for one child than another. You may need to try more than one fiber supplement in order to find the one that works the best for your child. Fiber supplements are particularly helpful in the treatment of children with occasional constipation who resist eating high fiber foods. Examples of fiber supplements are in Table 14.3.

Table 14.3 Fiber Supplements

Product	Form(s)*	Flavor	Grams/ Serving
Benefiber® (Natural)	powder	orange	3g
	chewable	no taste	3g
Metamucil® (Natural)	powder	orange pink lemonade berry	3g
	powder (clear)	no taste	5g
	wafers	apple crisp cinnamon	5g
Pedia-Lax® (Synthetic)	fiber gummies	assorted fruits	2g (each)

*Powders should be mixed in 6 to 8 oz of water.

Warning: When increasing fiber of any kind, do so gradually over a period of weeks in order to minimize the potential for gassiness, bloating, and cramps. This is especially true for children with severe constipation for whom these symptoms are often worse than for children with occasional constipation.

Liquid and fiber diary

Parents tend to overestimate how much fiber or liquid they think their child consumes in an average day.[2] For this reason, do not make any decisions regarding your child's dietary needs until you determine how much fiber or liquid he or she actually consumes. Filling out the "Weekly Record of Liquid and Dietary Fiber" (see Appendix) or an equivalent form is an efficient and accurate method for collecting this information.

Liquid and fiber diary instructions

In order to determine how many grams of fiber your child consumes in a day, you must look not only at the number of grams of dietary fiber indicated on a product's nutrition label, but also at the "serving size" required for that amount of fiber. Thus, on the record form you enter both the quantity (e.g., cups, slices) of food eaten and the grams of fiber shown on the nutrition label for that serving size.

Chapter Notes

1. Müller-Lissner, S.A., Kamm, M.A., Scarpignato, C., & Wald, A. (2005). Myths and misconceptions about functional constipation. *American Journal of Gastroenterology*, (100), 232–242.
2. American Dietetic Association. (2008). Position of the American dietetic association: Health implication of dietary fiber. *Journal of the American Dietetic Association*, 108, 1716–1731.
3. Institute of Medicine, National Academies. (2005). Dietary reference intakes for water, potassium, sodium, chloride, and sulfate. Washington D.C.: The National Academies Press. Retrieved from http://www.nal.usda.gov/fnic/DRI/DRI_Water/water_full_report.pdf, June, 2012.

Tummy Rubs for Pooping

15

Lower abdominal massage

Clinical research and case studies over the past ten years[1] have shown that lower abdominal massage, when done correctly on adults and children with ongoing constipation, can:

1. stimulate peristalsis
2. increase colonic transit time
3. increase bowel movement frequency

Abdominal massage is a positive adjunct to laxative therapy for many children, whether done by a qualified massage therapist, a parent, or the child. However, massage is not a stand-alone treatment for functional constipation and should only be done with accurate knowledge of the underlying anatomy.

Visual aid

A drawing of the large intestine (such as Figures 3.5 and 9.1) is useful for instructing parents and children about the anatomy of the abdomen. Use the visual aid to show how the large intestine or colon starts on the lower right side (the ascending section) and then goes up until it is parallel with the belly button. It then turns left and crosses horizontally just below the belly button (the transverse section) before turning down on the left side (the descending and sigmoid sections) on its way to the rectum.

Talk to your child about peristalsis and how it propels poop through the colon. Explain how peristalsis is triggered by the gastrocolic reflex which occurs within minutes of eating. Armed with this information, parents and children are better able to understand how a lower abdominal massage might help to relieve constipation.

Mild pressure

Massage is best described as applying mild to moderate hand pressure over the abdomen in the area of the transverse and descending colon. With young children, use a clockwise circular motion with the palm of the hand or the outside edge of the hand centered just below the child's belly button. Be sure to use a lubricant to reduce friction if the massage is done on bare skin.

Figure 15.1 Lower Abdominal Massage

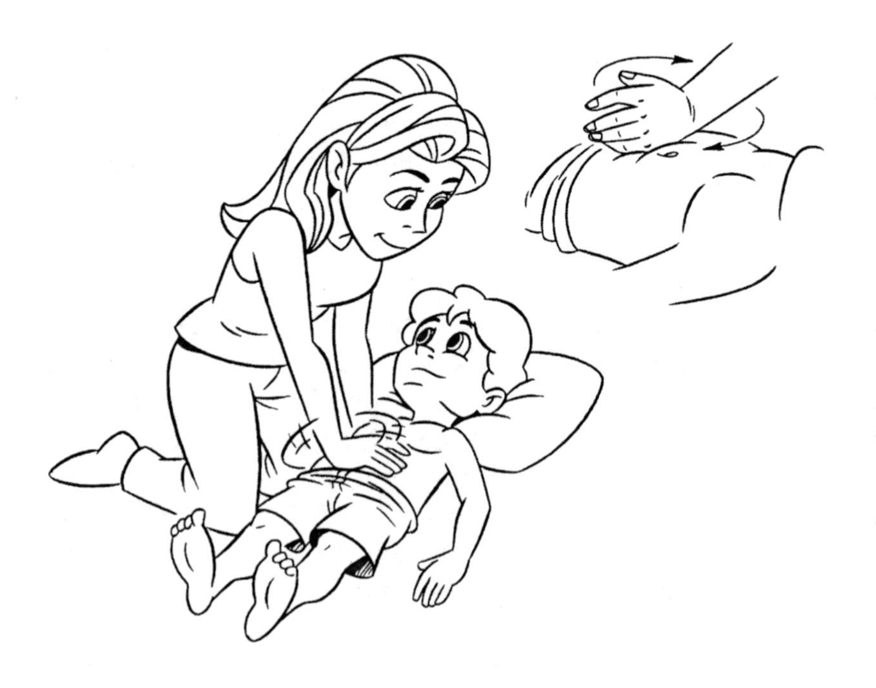

Stimulation and relaxation

The benefits of abdominal massage are most likely due to the combination of peristaltic stimulation and relaxation. Since peristalsis and relaxation are both conducive to passing stool, either the child or parent can do a brief abdominal massage while the child is sitting on the toilet to defecate. Whenever and wherever it is done, keep in mind that an abdominal massage can stimulate bowel sounds, flatulence and/or bowel movements.

Chapter Notes

1. Sinclair, M. (2011). The use of abdominal massage to treat functional constipation. *Journal of Bodywork and Movement Therapies*, 15(4), 436–445.

Bugs and Roots for Pooping

16

Probiotics and herbal therapy

Probiotics

Probiotics are living microorganisms, mostly bacteria, which are found in certain foods such as yogurt or fermented milk. These "bugs" are thought to increase the number of "good" bugs in our intestines. However, since there is little evidence that the balance of "good" and "bad" bacteria is abnormal in children who are constipated, the value of probiotics in the treatment of childhood constipation is unclear.[1]

Preliminary studies have shown that probiotics or combinations of probiotics may improve intestinal functioning and symptoms (e.g., transit time and frequency of bowel movements).[2,3] However, more research is needed to definitively determine whether probiotics are beneficial for children with functional constipation. If you decide to give your child a probiotic for constipation, it should be discontinued if there is no symptomatic improvement, or if your child's symptoms worsen. While probiotics are relatively safe, side effects may include "tummy aches," flatulence, and loose stools.[2]

Herbal therapy

Herbal therapies have been used since ancient times to treat a variety of disorders. Senna, the active ingredient in some stimulant laxatives, and rhubarb root are frequently used to treat constipation. For example, senna is commercially available in a stimulant laxative tea for adults and children. Many other herbal "medicines" such as hemp seed pills are generally safe and well tolerated. However, in spite of multiple studies, empirical evidence thus far has not confirmed the safety and efficacy of herbal products in the treatment of functional constipation.[4, 5]

Chapter Notes

1. Vandenplas, Y., & Benninga, M. (2009). Probiotics and functional gastrointestinal disorders in children. *Journal of Pediatric Gastroenterology and Nutrition*, 48 (Suppl. 2), S107–109.
2. DeMaria, N., Maier, D., & Ringel, Y. (2009-2010). Could probiotics help alleviate your functional gastrointestinal symptoms? (IFFG Handout #246), 1–4.
3. Bekkali, N., Bongers, M., Van den Berg, M.M., Liem, O., & Benninga, M.A. (2007). The role of a probiotics mixture in the treatment of childhood constipation. *Nutrition Journal*, 6, 17.
4. Cheng, C., Bian, Z., Wu, J., & Sung, J. (2011). Efficacy of Chinese herbal proprietary medicine (hemp seed pill) for functional constipation. *American Journal of Gastroenterology*, 106, 120–129.
5. Cheng, C., Bian, Z., & Wu, T. (2009). Systematic review of Chinese herbal medicine for functional constipation. *World Journal of Gastroenterology*, 15(39): 4886–4895.

Constipation Guide for Pediatric Healthcare Providers 17

A Recent Referral

I have a son who will turn nine in March of this year. He has had trouble with appropriate bathroom habits since the time we tried to toilet train him. He has consistently wet and soiled himself his entire life. He is very capable in every other aspect of his development. He is the oldest of three children (the other two have "normal" bathroom habits). He is very intelligent and socially aware for his age. He is in the "Highly Capable" program for gifted students in our school district and plays sports regularly.

We have tried everything we can think of to help him through this challenge. We have had him evaluated by several medical professionals and specialists. We have seen a psychiatrist. We have tried rewards and the removal of privileges. We have tried changes in diet and medication. NOTHING has helped. We have also tried just leaving him alone and hoping that if we backed off he might figure it out on his own.

I am very concerned about the social consequences he will soon face if we cannot help him to improve this situation. • ***Erin C.***

This family's long and frustrating search for help epitomizes the problem that this book—and especially this chapter—is intended to address: that most pediatric primary and specialty care providers have limited knowledge about and experience in treating functional constipation (encopresis). As a result, parents often go from one specialist to another in search of an explanation and treatment for their child's problem.

Part 1. Three keys to treatment success

The keys to successful treatment of functional constipation are to 1) treat the problem aggressively, 2) establish and maintain a collaborative provider-patient relationship throughout treatment, and 3) provide instruction in behavioral management strategies, thereby empowering parents and children to assume responsibility for implementing the treatment plan.

1. Treat aggressively

Laxatives must initially be dosed high enough to clean out the rectum. After the clean out, laxatives can then be titrated down (and sometimes back up) in order to achieve the desired goal of one to two soft but not watery bowel movements per day. The key is to stay aggressive. Primary care providers tend to undertreat constipation and withdraw laxatives too quickly rather than being sufficiently aggressive.[1, 2]

2. Collaborate and empower

A *collaborative* therapeutic relationship is essential when treating a functional GI disorder.[3] Unlike more typical provider-patient relationships associated with treating acute health problems, an active partnership with parents is essential to successfully managing the care of a child with encopresis over months and even years.

Operationally, this means allowing more time to listen and ask parents pertinent questions. It means being more available to parents via weekly office visits during the initial clean out and via office visits, telephone calls and e-mail thereafter. Often, when parents call in the midst of a crisis, what they want and need most is your confident reassurance that they are doing the right thing and that their child will get better.

By making parents integral members of the treatment team, you enlist their active participation in designing, implementing, and adjusting the treatment plan. You also give them the confidence to manage their child's care with increasingly less and, eventually, no assistance from you. I believe that our failure to teach and empower parents is one reason for the large number of children that remain symptomatic long after standard treatment for encopresis has ended.[1,4]

The following story, written by a parent, illustrates the value of a provider being readily available early in treatment while parents are still learning how to manage their child's treatment plan and be central players on the treatment team.

> **A Parent's Perspective on Accessibility**
> *Having an accessible care provider has made a big difference in the treatment of Miguel's constipation. When we first realized that Miguel had a problem, we went to see his pediatrician who is part of a large practice. He understood that Miguel's treatment was something we needed to monitor closely, but it was difficult to get in touch with him if a problem arose. I would need to call the doctor's office, leave a message for the nurse, and wait for her to call me back in a few hours. After giving the nurse further details, she would consult with the doctor when he was available and call me back with his advice a few hours later. If I still had concerns and wanted to speak with the doctor directly, I would need to wait until the end of the day for him to call me after he had finished seeing patients. If a problem arose after hours or*

on a weekend, my call would be routed through the answering service and there was very little chance that I would be able to speak to our doctor.

The specialist we are seeing now has provided a very different experience. He gave us his cell phone number from the start and has encouraged us to use it if needed. We were in contact every few days during Miguel's initial treatment. Miguel had been doing well but, at one point while we were on vacation, he started withholding again and things were clearly getting worse. I was having a difficult time managing the problem, but a short call to his doctor quickly got him back on track and we were all able to enjoy the rest of our trip.

A week after we returned, Miguel and I were looking over his poop chart, and I pointed out that he had had a big poop every single day for seven days without an enema. Miguel was so proud of what he had accomplished. He started jumping up and down and said, "Let's tell Dr. Tom!" I asked him if he wanted to wait until our appointment the next week or if he wanted to tell him right now. His immediate response was, "Right now!" I reminded him that Dr. Tom had told him that Miguel could call him on his cell phone if he had good news he wanted to share. Miguel (who has never been one for talking on the phone) called him right then to let him know how well he was doing. He was so excited to share his happy news, and the fact that he could do it in the moment really helped to foster their relationship.

• *Jennifer T.*

3. Include behavioral interventions

Treatment that combines medical management with instruction in behavioral intervention is significantly more successful than medical management alone.[5] It is one thing to tell a child to do something but it is another thing altogether to get the child to do it! Almost every child I have treated, regardless of age, has, at some point during their lengthy course of treatment, needed incentives to cooperate.

Most pediatric healthcare providers do not have the time and training to provide other than basic behavioral interventions.[6] This book contains helpful information for parents and providers about behavioral issues and incentive strategies (see chapter 13). Adding a trusted and qualified psychologist to the treatment team is also strongly recommended.

Parents and children may also benefit from participating in the internet program called "U-Can-Poop-Too" to learn about functional constipation and related behavioral management issues.[7]

Part 2. Evaluation and diagnosis

Routine questions about a child's bowel habits should be part of every pediatric visit. By asking about the average daily frequency, consistency and color, ease of pushing, and size of a child's stools, you can catch occasional constipation early and prevent its progression to functional constipation.

Childhood Constipation Questionnaire

If at any point during the evaluation you suspect constipation, or if a parent expresses concerns about constipation, have the parent complete the Childhood Constipation Questionnaire (CCQ) provided in the Appendix. The CCQ is useful in categorizing the level of severity as occasional or functional constipation. Take time to review parent's answers, checking for any omissions and clarifying responses. Most parents are not accustomed to answering questions about stool and bowel movements. The most common clinical signs associated with occasional and functional constipation are outlined in Table 17.1.

Table 17.1 Clinical Signs of Occasional and Functional Constipation

Occasional Constipation	Functional Constipation
4-5 bowel movements per week or "fewer than usual"	3 or fewer bowel movements per week
Sausage-shaped stools with cracked surfaces	Sausage/ball/pellet-shaped stools with cracked, lumpy surfaces
Brown to dark brown color	Dark brown to almost black color
Pushing harder and longer than usual	Frequent excessive straining
Uncomfortable bowel movements	Painful bowel movements
Large stools that "block the toilet"	Large stools that "block the toilet"
	Stool withholding
	Stool "accidents"

The constipation continuum

Parents find it helpful to learn that 1) a continuum exists from normal to occasional to functional constipation, 2) functional constipation (encopresis) is the most severe and persistent form of constipation, 3) early identification and treatment can shorten the course of treatment and prevent progression to functional constipation. Using the CCQ and the Bristol Stool Chart with parents is helpful in identifying where their child is along the continuum.

The Bristol Stool Chart

The Bristol Stool Chart[8] categorizes stool shape and consistency from small hard lumps to entirely liquid. The chart is a helpful assessment and instructional tool for both parents and providers.

Bristol Stool Chart

Type	Description
Type 1	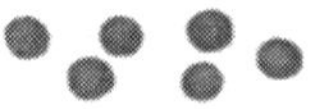 Separate hard lumps, like nuts (hard to pass)
Type 2	Sausage-shaped but lumpy
Type 3	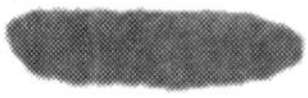 Like a sausage but with cracks on its surface
Type 4	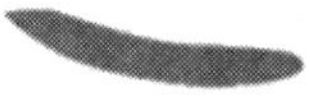 Like a sausage or snake, smooth and soft
Type 5	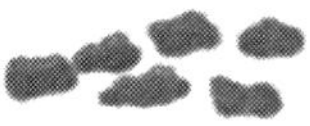 Soft blobs with clear-cut edges (passed easily)
Type 6	Fluffy pieces with ragged edges, a mushy stool
Type 7	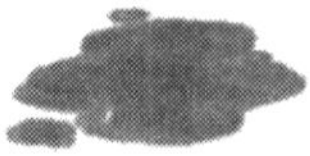 Watery, no solid pieces. **Entirely Liquid**

Functional constipation facts

In order to do a thorough diagnostic evaluation, pediatric providers should be knowledgeable about the physiology and behavioral manifestations of functional constipation.

Functional constipation starts when a child begins to involuntarily withhold stool following one or more painful bowel movements. As the excess stool accumulates in the rectum, and often higher up in the colon as well, the rectum begins to distend. Prolonged distention leads to rectal dysfunction.

Withholding ▶ Stretched rectum ▶ Rectal dysfunction

Withholding

Withholding begins as the purposeful retention of stool caused by the fear of pain. It is triggered by the feeling of urgency—the perceived need to pass stool. The act of withholding can quickly become an involuntary or habitual response depending on the child's temperament and the initial severity of pain. The more sensitive the child and the greater the pain, the more quickly withholding becomes involuntary and out of the child's control.

Withholding behaviors

- Clenching/squeezing the buttocks
- Extending or stiffening the body
- Crossing legs/ankles
- Excessive rocking or fidgeting
- Squatting with heel in crack of buttocks
- Hiding while defecating

Withholding is classified as complete or incomplete. Complete withholding occurs when a child passes almost no stool. Incomplete withholding occurs when a child passes varying amounts of stool but rarely evacuates completely. In both cases the retained stool accumulates and distends the rectum. However, the distention process is much slower for the incomplete withholder, sometimes taking months or years before the rectum is fully distended. Incomplete withholders are children who can be described as constipated, even though they may pass stool every day.

Rectal dysfunction

Prolonged stretching, in combination with continued rectal contractions, causes the walls of the rectum to become thicker and less elastic. Over time, this causes the stretch receptors in the inner wall of the rectum to lose their sensitivity to increasing amounts of stool.

Clinical indicators of rectal dysfunction

- Child does not feel "urgency"
- Defecations feel incomplete
- Stool incontinence
- Lower abdominal distention and "belly aches"
- Decreased appetite
- Nausea and vomiting
- Diurnal and nocturnal enuresis
- Lethargy
- Mood changes

Behaviors related to fear, hopelessness, and denial

The fear of pain which underlies habitual withholding will often expand or generalize to include sitting on the toilet or even to being in the bathroom to defecate. However, the fear does not typically prevent these children from using the toilet to urinate.

While some children with functional constipation do not cooperate because they just "don't want to," most children with functional constipation do not cooperate because they feel hopeless about getting better. They try to avoid or postpone being confronted with the problem by denying that it exists or by hiding the evidence. Nothing their parents or healthcare providers have done or told them to do has made their problem go away.

Clinical indicators of fear, hopelessness, and denial

- Not defecating while sitting on the toilet
- Only defecating in a diaper or Pull-up
- Not defecating in the bathroom
- Hiding to defecate (e.g., behind the sofa)
- Resisting/refusing to change soiled diaper/Pull-up
- Denying stool or wetting accidents
- Hiding soiled underwear/diaper/Pull-up

Diagnosing functional constipation

Functional constipation is a symptom-based disorder. A delay in diagnosing or starting treatment strengthens the habit of withholding and increases rectal stretching and rectal dysfunction.[4] If two or more of the objective criteria of functional constipation are present, particularly painful bowel movements, withholding and incontinence, an extensive diagnostic workup may be unnecessary. Most children with functional constipation do not have an underlying organic condition. (For example, Hirschsprung's disease is rarely a cause of functional constipation in older children.) A thorough history and physical exam are generally sufficient to make a diagnosis of functional constipation.[9]

Dyssynergic defecation

Some GI specialists believe that 25–50% of functional constipation is caused by *dyssynergic defecation*, a neuromuscular condition that causes "paradoxical contractions" of the external anal sphincter.[10] A paradoxical contraction is when the anal sphincter does not contract during pushing and thereby prevents the passage of stool. In clinical practice, constipation caused by neuromuscular dysfunction is rare, especially in children.[11] In the vast majority of cases, the involuntary contraction of the external anal sphincter is a *learned* response. It is not due to neuromuscular dysfunction per se.

While there may be some children who withhold because of an underlying neuromuscular abnormality, the most commonly used diagnostic and treatment procedures are so invasive and generally unavailable, that most GI specialists recommend first trying the standard treatments for functional constipation described in this book. If a child does not respond to standard treatment, a relatively non-invasive Sitzmark Study[12] can be extremely helpful in distinguishing stool withholding from dyssynergic defecation.

Part 3. Treatment of functional constipation

Goals

There are two main **treatment goals** for functional constipation.

1. ***Eliminate withholding and excessive stool retention*** to allow time for the rectum to shrink back to its normal size and regain its tone, elasticity and stool sensitivity.
2. ***Educate parents about functional constipation, the use of laxatives, and behavioral strategies*** to empower them to manage their child's ongoing care with decreasing professional assistance.

Laxatives

Whether administered orally or rectally, laxatives are a treatment necessity. Therefore, providing parents with accurate information about laxative use is extremely important. Parents' most common concerns have to do with the higher-than-usual dosages and the longer-than-usual length of time that laxatives must be used to successfully treat functional constipation.

Information you provide about these issues may conflict with what parents read or hear elsewhere. For example, you will be educating parents that the water retention laxative, polyethylene glycol (PEG), is safe and can be taken almost indefinitely. However, some PEG labels say, "Use no more than seven days." You will be educating parents that treating functional constipation often requires long-term use of stimulant laxatives. However, the label on a common product says, "Stop use and ask a doctor if you need to use for more than one week." You may be telling parents to give their child large quantities of mineral oil, especially during cleanouts. However, parents often fear that long-term use of mineral oil will cause vitamin deficiency. It is no wonder that parents become concerned and confused!

Laxative facts

Healthcare specialists who have studied the use of laxatives and who have successfully treated large numbers of children with functional constipation agree on the following:

- Functional constipation should be diagnosed quickly and treated aggressively with oral and/or rectal laxatives in sufficient quantity to evacuate the rectum and other sections of the colon when necessary.[1,2]
- Stopping laxatives too soon is the most common cause of relapse.[13]
- Stimulant laxatives are not harmful to the colon. They can be used safely for whatever length of time treatment requires. Stimulant laxatives do not cause *cathartic colon* or *dependency*.[14,15]
- Stimulant laxatives can be combined with bulk or osmotic laxatives in sufficient amounts to soften the stool or they can be used alone, according to clinical circumstances. The dose of such agents should be titrated to effect.[14]
- The fear of vitamin deficiency is unfounded. Studies have never shown any noticeable impact on the levels of fat-soluble vitamins in children or adults taking mineral oil even for long periods of time.[16]

Laxative tips

1. No standard maintenance dose exists for children with functional constipation. Some children respond well to very small doses (e.g., ½ tsp per day) while others need much higher doses (e.g., 10 tsp per day). Do not dose powdered laxatives by the "cap." Advise parents to use measuring spoons. For reference, one cap of polyethylene glycol (PEG) is equivalent to approximately 5 measured teaspoons.

   The following parent's story illustrates how sensitive some children can be to minor laxative adjustments.

Sensitive to a PEG Laxative

My 5 ½-year-old daughter, Sophia, has been dealing with encopresis since she was a baby. In the past, we had lowered or raised her dose of laxative using the cap on almost a daily basis, depending on her "output" or lack thereof. It seemed that whenever we changed her dose, her bowels became too loose or too hard. We now know that Sophia is very sensitive to her PEG laxative and that we have to make changes using measuring spoons. A dose of 4 teaspoons a day works consistently with Sophia's body. • ***Erin P.***

2. Be sure to advise parents at the outset that multiple dose adjustments may be necessary in order to achieve the desired goal of daily, medium to large, and soft but not watery, bowel movements throughout the course of treatment.

3. Advise parents at the outset that a combination of water retention and stimulant laxatives is often necessary to achieve the desired goal.

Follow-up is critical

One of the most serious mistakes by healthcare providers that impacts treatment outcomes is inadequate follow-up with parents, particularly during and after the initial cleanout. Be careful not to assume that parents completely understand what they have been told. Don't assume that they will call if they have questions or encounter an unexpected situation. Some parents have continued to give their children a PEG laxative years after it was first recommended by a pediatrician. Some do so because they think they have been instructed to give it *indefinitely* while others continue because their child's constipation returns when they try to stop. Follow-up visits or telephone contact can prevent these mistakes.

Follow-up visits and telephone contact

Scheduling brief, weekly in-office follow-up visits is recommended from the beginning of Step 2 and continuing on to Step 3 until an efficacious laxative protocol has been established. Subsequent meetings are usually done by telephone at one- to two-month intervals from the middle of Step 3 to the end of Step 5. I have found that most parents, when asked to call the office by a certain date in order to go over their child's WLSR data, do so faithfully. If they forget, I will call them.

The content of most follow-up visits, either in-office or telephone, includes: 1) a review of the WLSR data; 2) making any necessary laxative adjustments; 3) trouble-shooting incentive or behavioral programs; 4) giving reassurance that the treatment plan is working—even if it appears to be progressing by two steps forward, one step backward.

Six-Step Treatment Program

Treating functional constipation is more than just a cleanout. It involves ending withholding and allowing time for the rectum to shrink back to its normal size. Six steps are required to achieve these results. The length of time required for each step varies widely from child to child. Average times are listed in Table 17.2.

Table 17.2 Six-Step Treatment Program for Functional Constipation

Steps	Average Completion Time
1. Educate the family	1-3 months
2. Empty the rectum	1-4 days
3. End withholding	3-6 months
4. Shrink the rectum	3-12 months
5. Withdraw laxative(s)	1-3 months
6. Remain vigilant	6-12 months

■ Step 1. Educate the family (1-3 months)

Parents and children often find it difficult to understand the complexities of functional constipation. Pertinent information needs to be repeated and questions answered over a period of weeks and months before they finally "get it." The "demystification" of functional constipation is absolutely essential for long term treatment success.

Parents find it hard to believe that their child does not have an organic disorder when they see their child in pain day after day because he or she cannot poop. They assume there must be another more serious medical or psychological reason for the condition. Anticipate these concerns and be patient and confident in your educational response. In my experience, parents and children who can explain functional constipation and its treatment have better treatment outcomes than those who cannot. See chapter 9. The ABCs of Constipation, for ideas on how to explain functional constipation to parents and children and answer common questions.

Frequently-asked questions

1. What is functional constipation?
2. What causes functional constipation?
3. How dangerous is functional constipation?
4. Can functional constipation be cured?

Visual aids of the GI tract (e.g., Figures 3.1 and 9.1) are especially helpful for maintaining attention and enhancing learning.

Data collection

Ask parents to fill out a Weekly Laxative and Stool Record (WLSR) every day from the beginning of Step 1 until the end of Step 5 and to bring completed records with them to every visit. Use of this or an equivalent data collection tool avoids problems associated with long-term recall and provides a quick way of assessing progress over time. Records can be sent electronically to healthcare providers for telephone follow up. As treatment progresses and parents learn from their healthcare provider how to interpret data on the daily records, most parents become adept at making treatment changes on their own. The WLSR in the Appendix may be enlarged and copied for use by parents.

What does the Weekly Laxative and Stool Record (WLSR) tell us?

Daily tracking is the only way of knowing whether the treatment plan is being implemented correctly and whether the laxative protocol needs to be altered. What we want to see in the data is stool consistency that is routinely soft but not watery, stool color that is mostly light brown, and stool size that is mostly medium to large.

It Seemed a Bit Excessive

At first, the Weekly Laxative and Stool Record we were asked to keep for our daughter seemed a bit excessive. I did not think that I would have the time to write down every little thing, and I felt overwhelmed. But now that we have been doing it for ten weeks, we can see how beneficial it really is. Without the record, I am certain that we would over- or underestimate our daughter's stool frequency and output. Having an accurate history helps us to see when detrimental stool patterns are starting to develop, which allows us to make laxative adjustments before the pattern has gone on too long. The record helps us do a better job of celebrating and rewarding our daughter's efforts. I can also say, without a doubt, that the record has kept us on schedule with our daughter's poop medicines. It is a constant reminder and we hardly ever miss a dose. At this point, it's an integral part of our daily routine. • ***Brynne B.***

What do stool accidents tell us?

The frequency and consistency of stool accidents provide another way of determining whether the recommended laxative and/or its dosage are correct. If stool is still dry (e.g., dark brown sausages with cracks) four to five days after starting a laxative, the dose usually needs to be increased or the choice of laxative changed. If stool is loose or watery at this point, the dose needs to be lowered.

■ Step 2. Empty the rectum (1-4 days)

In most but not all cases of functional constipation, an excessive amount of stool builds up in the rectum. Large quantities of stool may also be found higher up in the colon. Some children have excess stool as far back as the ascending colon. The presence of an excessive amount of stool in the colon can be determined by digital rectal exam, lower abdominal palpation or lower abdominal x-ray.

The likelihood of rectal distention increases the longer this accumulating mass of stool remains in the rectum. Since rectal or colonic distention is the physiological genesis of functional constipation, the immediate removal of the stool mass is essential. The high doses of laxatives necessary for effective cleanouts may also cause uncontrollable leaking. For this reason, cleanouts are typically best done on weekends when a child is not in school or daycare.

To clean out excess stool quickly, use one or more of the following laxative choices:

1. Higher than usual doses of orally administered water retention laxatives
2. Lubricating laxatives such as mineral oil
3. Rectally administered laxatives (enemas or suppositories)

Leaking caused by laxatives

At the end of a cleanout, the laxative dose is usually decreased. If a child continues to leak stool, do not immediately conclude that his or her rectum must still be impacted and that the dose should be kept high or increased further. In fact, the high dose of laxative(s) used in cleanouts often causes continued leaking. By maintaining or increasing the dose, you may cause the child to leak even more. Post-cleanout digital rectal exams or lower abdominal x-rays are helpful for determining whether continued leaking is due to excess stool or laxatives.

■ Step 3. End withholding (3-6 months)

It is important to accept that [treatment] is likely to be protracted and subject to disappointing relapses that demoralize all those involved.[13]

Once the stool mass has been removed, the next challenge is to find the laxative or combination of laxatives that, along with sitting and pushing incentives, will enable a child to push out one or two medium-to-large bowel movements a day. Finding the ideal dose can be frustrating due to the unintended consequences of dose adjustments that may be too low or too high. Bowel movements must be sufficiently soft to pass through the anal canal and the external anal sphincter without causing pain or discomfort.

The uninterrupted repetition of comfortable bowel movements will gradually extinguish a child's learned association of pain with urgency, along with the related habit of withholding.

Follow-up during Step 3

Continue to follow up as planned and respond as quickly as possible to crisis phone calls or requests for an in-office appointment.

■ Step 4. Shrink the rectum (3-12 months)

During this period the rectum regains its normal tone, elasticity and sensitivity. This is also the time when stool accidents gradually decrease in size and frequency. There is no way to determine whether or when the rectum has fully recovered. In fact, it may be that the rectum never fully recovers.[17] This may account for the fact that treatment follow-up studies show that almost 40% of children continue to have symptoms of functional constipation three and one-half to twelve years after completing treatment.[4,18] One of the aims of this book is to decrease these discouraging percentages.

Follow up during Step 4

From the point of view of the child and his/her parents, this stage of treatment is probably the most difficult because there is no way for them to know if or when the rectum has recovered. Follow up during this step is mainly to provide praise and encouragement and to decide when to begin Step 5.

■ Step 5. Withdraw laxatives (1-3 months)

This is the step that parents and children eagerly look forward to because they want to be done with the laxatives as quickly as possible. Nevertheless, laxatives must be withdrawn slowly because, if stopped too soon or too abruptly, withholding may recur and laxatives will again be necessary.

How to withdraw laxatives

Err on the side of caution when advising parents to start withdrawing laxatives. Withdrawing slowly is better than risking the return of withholding and rectal distention.

1. Withdraw stimulant laxatives first.
2. Lower doses very gradually, e.g., by ½ tsp.
3. Wait four to five days between dose reductions to assess effect.
4. Return to the previous higher dose if stools begin to dry or if the frequency of bowel movements decreases.

5. Once bowel movements have normalized, continue on the previous dose for at least three weeks before trying another dose reduction.

■ Step 6. Remain vigilant (6-12 months)

Once a child is having daily bowel movements and has been off all laxatives for an extended period of time, parents understandably think they no longer need to pay attention to their child's bowel movements. This is definitely not true. Children with a history of functional constipation are at risk of becoming constipated again. Therefore, you should strongly advise parents to check frequently to see that their child is continuing to have daily (or almost daily) bowel movements and that their stool is normal in size and consistency.

Expected treatment outcomes

In my experience, adherence to this Six-Step Program will eliminate stool withholding and incontinence in most children with functional constipation. Maintenance laxative and behavioral treatment, managed primarily by parents, is still necessary in almost all cases until the child feels normal bowel urgency and laxatives have been successfully withdrawn. The length of time between the completion of Steps 3 (stop withholding) and 4 (shrink the rectum) and the completion of Step 5 (withdraw laxatives) varies considerably, depending on the initial severity of constipation, the child's age and temperament and parental persistence.

Chapter Notes

1. Borowitz, S. M., Cox, D. J., Kovatchev, B., Ritterbrand, L. M., Sheen, J., Sutphen, J. (2005). Treatment of childhood constipation by primary care physicians: efficacy and predictors of outcome. *Pediatrics*, 115 (4): 873–877.
2. DiLorenzo C. Personal communication with Dr. Carlo DiLorenzo, Director, Motility Center, Children's Hospital of Columbus, OH, Professor of Pediatrics, The Ohio State

University, Columbus, OH, 2011.

3. Thompson, W.G. (2008). Understanding the irritable gut: The functional gastrointestinal disorders. McLean, VA: Degnon Associates, Inc.
4. Loening-Baucke, V. (1993). Constipation in early childhood: Patient characteristics, treatment and long-term follow up. *Gut*, 1400–1404.
5. McGrath, M. L., Mellon, M. W., and Murphy, L. (2000). Empirically supported treatments in pediatric psychology: constipation and encopresis. *Journal of Pediatric Psychology,* 25, 225–254.
6. Ritterbrand, L. M., Cox, D. J., Kovatchev, B., Borowitz, S., et al. (2003). An internet intervention as adjunctive therapy for pediatric encopresis. *Journal of Consulting and Clinical Psychology.* 71 (5): 910–917.
7. Ritterband, L. M., Ardalan, K., Thorndike, F. P., Magee, J. C., Saylor, D. K., Cox, D. J., Sutphen, J. L. & Borowitz, S. M. (2008). Real world use of an internet intervention for pediatric encopresis. *Journal of Medical Internet Research*, 10 (2), e16. doi:10.2196/jmir.1081
8. Lewis, S.J. and Heaton, K.W. (1997). Stool form scale as a useful guide to intestinal transit time. *Skandinavian Journal of Gastronenterology,* 32(9): 920-24.
9. Brandt, L. J., Prather, C. M., Quigley, E. M., Schiller, L. R., Schoenfeld, P., & Talley, N. J. (2005). Systematic review on the management of functional constipation in North America. *American Journal of Gastroenterology*, 100 (S1), S1–S22. doi: 10.1111/j.1572-0241.2005.50613.x
10. Rao, S. (2010). Dyssynergic defecation: Questions and answers about a common cause of functional constipation. IFFGD Fact Sheet No. 237, 1–4.
11. Pisharody U. Personal communication with Dr. Uma Pisharody, pediatric gastroenterologist, pediatric specialty care, Swedish Medical Center, Seattle, WA, 2012.
12. Children's Hospital of the Kings Daughters. Sitzmark Study:

Healthy Facts. n.d., Retrieved 5/20/12, from http://www.chkd.org/HealthLibrary/Facts/Content.aspx?pageid=0395

13. Clayden, G. S. (1992). Management of functional constipation. *Archives of Disease in Childhood*, 67, 340–344.
14. Wald A. (2003). Is chronic use of stimulant laxatives harmful to the colon? [Clinical Reviews]. *Journal of Clinical Gastroenterology,* 36(5), 386–389.
15. Müller-Lissner, S. A., Kamm, M. A., Scarpignato, C., & Wald, A. (2005). Myths and misconceptions about functional constipation. *American Journal of Gastroenterology*, 100, 232–242.
16. Levy, J. & Volpert, D. (2005). Know thy laxatives: A parent's guide to the successful management of chronic functional constipation in infants and children. IFFGD Fact Sheet No.828, 1–4.
17. Loening-Baucke, V. (1984). Abnormal rectoanal function in children recovered from functional constipation and encopresis. *Gastroenterology*, 87 (6), 1299–1304.
18. Loening-Baucke, V. (2002). Functional fecal retention in childhood. *Practical Gastroenterology*, 25, 213–221.

Resources

Organization

International Foundation for Functional Gastrointestinal Disorders (IFFGD)
P.O. Box 170864, Milwaukee, WI 53217-8076
Toll-free Telephone: 888-964-2001
www.iffgd.org

Books

Drossman, D. A., Corazziari, E., Delvaux, M., Spiller, R. C., Talley, N. J., Thompson, W. G., Whitehead, W. E., Eds. (2006). *Rome III: The Functional Gastrointestinal Disorders*. McLean, VA: Degnon Associates, Inc.

Hodges, S. J. (2012). *It's No Accident*. Guilford, CT: Globe Pequot Press.

Smith, D. P. (2004). *Overcoming Childhood Bladder and Bowel Problems*. Knoxville, TN: Potty MD.

Thompson, W. G. (2008). *Understanding the Irritable Gut*. McLean, VA: Degnon Associates, Inc.

Websites

www.ucanpooptoo.com

An online program for pediatric encopresis

www.theinsandoutsofpoop.com

Data collection forms and visual aids for evaluating and educating families about functional constipation

Appendix

CHILDHOOD CONSTIPATION QUESTIONNAIRE

Name:________________________________Date:________

Directions: Circle "yes" or "no" for each answer.
Scoring: Count the number of "Yes" responses. A score of 5-10 may be indicative of "occasional constipation." A score over 10 may be indicative of "functional constipation."

Frequency	1. Is the frequency of your child's bowel movement (on average):		
	a. 6-7 times or more per week?..................	Yes	No
	b. 4-5 times per week?................................	Yes	No
	c. 1-3 times per week?................................	Yes	No
	d. less than 1 time per week?......................	Yes	No
Consistency	2. Does the shape and surface of your child's stools (on average) look like:		
	a. balls, pellets with cracks?........................	Yes	No
	b. log, sausage with lumps?..........................	Yes	No
	c. log, sausage with cracks?.........................	Yes	No
	d. banana, snake with smooth surface?	Yes	No
	e. soft blobs, stringy?..................................	Yes	No
	f. applesauce, pudding, mushy?..................	Yes	No
	g. diarrhea, liquid?.......................................	Yes	No
	3. Is the color of your child's stools (on average):		
	a. golden brown to brown?........................	Yes	No
	b. dark brown?...	Yes	No
	c. very dark brown?.....................................	Yes	No
	d. almost black?..	Yes	No
	4. Have your child's stools ever blocked or "plugged up" the toilet?	Yes	No
Pushing/ Straining	5. Does your child have to strain (push very hard) to have a bowel movement?	Yes	No
Pain/ Discomfort	6. Does your child have uncomfortable or painful bowel movements?	Yes	No
	7. Does your child complain of stomach discomfort or bellyaches?	Yes	No
Avoidance/ Resistance	8. Has your child ever expressed a fear of the toilet?	Yes	No
	9. Does your child resist sitting on the toilet to have a bowel movement?	Yes	No
	10. Does your child resist going into the bathroom to have a bowel movement?	Yes	No

Continued

Withholding	11. Does your child try to keep him/herself from passing stool?	Yes	No
	12. Have you ever seen your child in any of the following positions?		
	a. Squeezing legs tightly together while sitting on the toilet..	Yes	No
	b. Squeezing or crossing legs while standing	Yes	No
	c. Squatting/kneeling with heel of one foot pressed between his/her buttocks......................	Yes	No
	13. Does your child go some place other than the bathroom to have a bowel movement?	Yes	No
	If yes, circle all that apply.		
	a. Bedroom		
	b. Living room		
	c. Behind couch		
	d. Other:		
Accidents/ Stool Incontinence	14. Does your child ever say that he/she does not feel the need to have a bowel movement?	Yes	No
	15. Does your child ever have bowel "accidents" or soiling of his/her underwear?	Yes	No
	16. Do any of these terms best describe your child's "accidents?"		
	a. Just a stain..	Yes	No
	b. Smear (thin stain)......................................	Yes	No
	c. Small and loose..	Yes	No
	d. Large pieces..	Yes	No
	e. Full bowel movement................................	Yes	No
	f. Extremely variable......................................	Yes	No
	g. Mixed with urine..	Yes	No
	17. Does your child have bowel movements while playing or watching TV/video games or using the computer?	Yes	No
	18. Does your child have "accidents" while asleep at night?	Yes	No
	19. Does your child wet his/her underwear/ clothing during the day?	Yes	No
	20. Does your child wet the bed at night?	Yes	No
Denial/ Hiding/ Resistance	21. Does your child deny having had a bowel movement?	Yes	No
	22. Does your child hide soiled or wet underwear?	Yes	No
Score	Total number of "yes" responses: _____		

Adapted with permission from Encopresis Evaluation System (unpublished) developed by Drs. Melvin D. Levine and Ronald Barr.

FIBER CONTENT OF SELECTED FOODS

FOOD	SERVING SIZE	DIETARY FIBER (g)*	SOLUBLE FIBER (g)*	INSOLUBLE FIBER (g)*
Cereal				
Fiber One (Bran)	½ cup	14.0	1.0	13.0
Fiber One (with raisins)	1 cup	11.0	3.0	8.0
All Bran (extra fiber)	½ cup	13.0	1.0	12.0
All Bran (original)	½ cup	10.0	1.0	9.0
All Bran (Yogurt Bites)	1 ¼ cup	10.0	1.0	9.0
All Bran (Wheat Flakes)	¾ cup	6.0	1.0	5.0
Raisin Bran	1 cup	8.0	1.0	7.0
Shredded Wheat'n Bran	1 ¼ cup	8.0	1.0	7.0
Shredded Wheat (Mini)	30 pieces	6.0	1.0	5.0
Cheerios	1 cup	3.0	1.0	2.0
oatmeal (dry)	½ cup	4.0	2.0	2.0
Breads				
whole Grain	1 slice	2.9	0.4	2.5
French bread	1 slice	1.0	0.4	0.6
whole wheat bread	1 slice	1.6	1.3	0.3
rye bread	1 slice	2.7	1.4	1.3
wheat Bagel	1 medium	3.0	1.0	2.0
white bread	1 slice	0.5	0.2	0.3
Pasta/Rice				
spaghetti (cooked)	½ cup	0.8	0.0	0.8
white rice (cooked)	½ cup	0.5	0.5	0.0
brown rice (cooked)	½ cup	1.3	1.3	0.0
Legumes/Lentils				
chick peas	½ cup	5.0	1.0	4.0
kidney beans (cooked)	½ cup	4.5	0.5	4.0
pinto beans (cooked)	½ cup	7.4	5.5	1.9
lima beans (cooked)	½ cup	1.4	0.2	1.2
white beans (cooked)	½ cup	4.2	0.4	3.8
lentils (cooked)	2/3 cup	4.5	0.6	3.9
Fruits				
apple	1 medium	5.7	4.2	1.5

FOOD	SERVING SIZE	DIETARY FIBER (g)*	SOLUBLE FIBER (g)*	INSOLUBLE FIBER (g)*
banana	1 medium	2.8	2.1	0.7
blackberries	½ cup	3.7	0.7	3.0
kiwi	1 large	3.1	2.4	0.7
orange	1 medium	4.4	2.6	1.8
pear	1 medium	2.9	1.8	1.1
raspberries	½ cup	4.2	3.8	0.4
prunes (dried)	3 medium	1.7	1.0	1.2
figs	3 small	5.3	3.0	2.3
strawberries	¾ cup	2.4	0.9	1.5
Vegetables				
artichoke (cooked)	1 medium	6.5	4.7	1.8
broccoli	1 stalk	2.7	1.3	1.4
corn	2/3 cup	1.6	0.2	1.4
peas (cooked)	½ cup	5.2	2.0	3.2
potato (with skin)	1 medium	2.9	1.7	1.2
parsnips (cooked)	½ cup	2.9	1.7	1.2
green peas (cooked)	2/3 cup	3.9	0.6	3.3
Snacks/Bars				
popcorn	6 cups	5.6	1.6	4.0
Fiber One (Chewy)	1 bar	9.0	-	-
Fiber One (Brownie)	1 brownie	5.0	-	-

*Grams per serving

Note that fiber content can vary between brands.

Sources:

http://www.fatfreekitchen.com/soluble-fiber-foods-list.html (Retrieved 12/12/2011)

http://www.healthhype.com/list-of-high-fiber-foods-soluble-and-insoluble-fiber-chart.html (Retrieved 12/12/2011)

http://www.mayoclinic.com/health/high-fiber-foods/NUoo582/METHOD=print (Retrieved 12/8/2011)

http://www.wehealny.org/healthinfo/dietaryfiber/fibercontentchart.html (Retrieved 12/8/2011)

WEEKLY RECORD OF LIQUID AND DIETARY FIBER

Name: ____________________ Week of: ____________

FOOD GROUP (Qty)	**Sunday**		**Monday**		**Tuesday**		**Wednesday**		**Thursday**		**Friday**		**Saturday**	
	Qty	Grams	Qty	Grams	Qty	Grams	Qty	Grams	Qty	Grams	Qty	Grams	Qty	Grams
cereal (cups)														
bread (slices)														
grains (cups)														
legumes (cups)														
fruit (# or size)														
vegetables (cups)														
other														
Total Dietary Fiber (Grams)														
Total Liquid (8 oz cups)														

WEEKLY LAXATIVE AND STOOL RECORD

Name:																					
	Sunday			Monday			Tuesday			Wednesday			Thursday			Friday			Saturday		
Date: Year Month: Day:																					
Laxative(s):																					
#1 Dose:																					
Time:																					
#2 Dose:																					
Time:																					
Stool Record	#			#			#			#			#			#			#		
	1	2	3	1	2	3	1	2	3	1	2	3	1	2	3	1	2	3	1	2	3
1. Time of bowel movement																					
2. Shape and edges *(Check one)*																					
Balls, pellets/cracks																					
Log, sausage/lumpy																					
Log, sausage/cracks																					
Banana, snake/smooth																					
Soft blobs, stringy																					
Applesauce, pudding, mushy																					
Diarrhea, liquid																					
3. Color *(Check one)*																					
Light, golden brown																					
Brown, dark brown																					
4. Size *(Enter S/M/L)*																					
Small/Medium/Large																					
5. Accident(s) *(Number per day)*																					

Bristol Stool Chart

Type	Description
Type 1	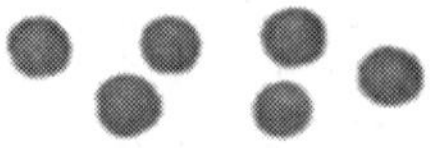 Separate hard lumps, like nuts (hard to pass)
Type 2	Sausage-shaped but lumpy
Type 3	Like a sausage but with cracks on its surface
Type 4	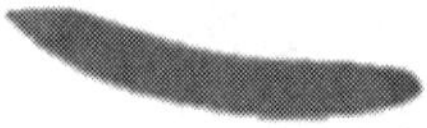 Like a sausage or snake, smooth and soft
Type 5	Soft blobs with clear-cut edges (passed easily)
Type 6	Fluffy pieces with ragged edges, a mushy stool
Type 7	Watery, no solid pieces. **Entirely Liquid**

Index

ABOUT THE AUTHOR

Dr. Thomas R. DuHamel is a clinical child psychologist in private practice with the Associates in Behavior and Child Development, ABCD Inc, in Seattle, Washington. He is a Clinical Associate Professor in the Department of Psychiatry and Behavioral Sciences at the University of Washington School of Medicine. Dr. DuHamel graduated from Brown University and earned his doctorate in clinical psychology at the University of Massachusetts at Amherst. He completed a post doctoral residency in the Department of Medical Psychology at the University of Oregon Medical School in Portland and was formerly Chief Psychologist at Seattle Children's Hospital.

Dr. DuHamel is married with two children and a very precious granddaughter.

CPSIA information can be obtained at www.ICGtesting.com
Printed in the USA
BVOW041846150812

297986BV00004B/11/P